Kate Holmes 24.1.91.

Domiciliary Terminal Car

C000058969

Domiciliary Terminal Care

A HANDBOOK FOR DOCTORS AND NURSES

Derek Doyle OBE FRCPEd FRCGP

CHURCHILL LIVINGSTONE
EDINBURGH LONDON MELBOURNE AND NEW YORK 1987

CHURCHILL LIVINGSTONE
Medical Division of Longman Group UK Limited

Distributed in the United States of America by
Churchill Livingstone Inc., 1560 Broadway, New York,
N.Y. 10036, and by associated companies, branches
and representatives throughout the world.

First published 1987

ISBN   0-443-03697-7

British Library Cataloguing in Publication Data
Doyle, Derek
    Domiciliary terminal care: a handbook for doctors
    and nurses.
    1. Terminal care. 2. Home nursing. I. Title.
    I. Title
    649.8   R726.8

Library of Congress Cataloging in Publication Data
Doyle, Derek.
    Domiciliary terminal care.

    Bibliography: p.
    1. Terminal care. 2. Home nursing. I. Title.
[DNLM: 1. Home Care Services. 2. Terminal Care.
WB 310 D754d]
RT87.T45D69 1987   616'.029   87–751

Produced by Longman Singapore Publishers (Pte) Ltd.
Printed in Singapore.

Contents

Introduction

There are a few indisputable facts about the terminally ill which, in themselves, are sufficient justification for this handbook.

Most of their final year of life is spent at home under the care of their family doctors and community nurses. Admittedly only about 30% die at home in the cities and 40% in the country districts and many have several periods of hospital care before the final admission. Nevertheless, close on 90% of the final year of life is spent at home.

Equally important is the frequently observed and recorded fact that more than half of all patients interviewed in different studies had expressed the wish to remain at home as long as possible and, if it is feasible, to die at home.

Consequently it is at home that most of the problems and challenges are met, whether physical, psychological or nursing problems or family difficulties. It falls to the members of the primary care team to anticipate some and treat others. It is to them that relatives will turn, not only whilst the patient is still alive but, in the best traditions of family practice, in the months and years which follow.

That most colleagues working in the community recognize this and actively set out to improve their skills is amply demonstrated by their attendance at the many special courses and conferences on 'Care of the Dying' and by the encouragement the author has received in preparing this handbook.

A few words of explanation about the book are appropriate here. It is not a reference book to which one can turn for everything which is known on the subject, supported by extensive reference to published works. Neither is it intended as an erudite textbook. The author assumes that all who read it are clinically experienced, know sufficient basic pharamacology and therapeutics to practise domiciliary terminal care, and are already familiar with the types of problems experienced in providing such care for the terminally ill.

Though guidelines may be set down there can seldom be hard and fast rules when caring for the dying. All that the author is offering is advice based on his own experience in general practice in Britain and abroad, enhanced by additional knowledge and insight from many years in a hospice unit which operates a large domiciliary advisory service for colleagues in primary care teams.

Advice, suggestions and encouragement have come from hospice doctors, community colleagues, patients and families, to all of whom the author records his indebtedness. Where ideas are good the credit can go to them; where faults and mistakes are found, the blame must fall on the author.

Throughout the book the male gender is generally used, for convenience and brevity rather than chauvinism, without any intended insult to female colleagues or patients. It is the hope of the author that the handbook will bring new ideas to some, encouragement to others, and the quality of care they so richly deserve to all whom we serve, in town or country.

The author would record his indebtedness to patients, colleagues and publishers and, in particular, to Dr T F Benton (Consultant Physician, St Columba's Hospice) and Mrs Irene Turnbull for her unfailing patience in typing and preparing the manuscript.

1

Pain control

Probably only those who have experienced chronic pain have any idea of what it means. It is not so much its intensity as the fact that it may go on for days or weeks or for ever, which terrifies people. They wake up in the morning and their first thoughts are whether they have pain, how bad it will be that day, how long they may be able to bear it without resorting to drugs, how much it will affect what they hope to do, and whether those who look after them — family or professionals — will believe them and take them seriously. They tell us that pain controls their lives and often do so in terms which may easily make the professional wonder if there is a neurotic element.

Chronic pain is so different from acute pain though the latter is often much more severe. Fortunately acute pain is easily described and recognized by the patient as well as his attendants, as helpful in coming to a diagnosis. As a result it commands attention and, hopefully, speedy relief. This is exemplified in the pain of myocardial infarction, renal or biliary colic, pleurisy or fractures. Sadly most doctors and nurses are taught more about acute than chronic pain and many not only feel helpless to relieve chronic pain but often display interest bordering on apathy. The reasons are obvious.

Chronic pain is, after a while, poorly described by the patient until finally it is often borne in silence. He had to be urged to describe it and confidently shown that there are means of relieving it. Any apparent loss of professional interest or enthusiasm is soon misinterpreted by the patient as disbelief in his suffering or a silent affirmation that no relief is in fact available. He becomes morose and withdrawn, takes no interest in his surroundings and can easily be mis-diagnosed as suffering from depression which seems so logical if the patient is terminally ill.

A good rule, particularly with cancer patients, is to assume they have pain until proved otherwise. It is equally useful to remember that with the terminally ill, 'No pain reported' means no more, no less than that — if he has pain it was not reported! It does not mean, as it would with an acute condition, that in fact he has no pain.

The fact that only about 60–70% of cancer patients ever suffer pain and even fewer of those with cardiac, respiratory or neurological conditions does not stop our patients expecting it, dreading it, or needing very positive professional help and support. The layman's notion that cancer equals death with uncontrollable pain, has unfortunately some foundation as many studies have shown that up to one-third of patients do die with poorly controlled pain. This need not happen any more than a patient need be sedated unnecessarily just because he is dying.

PRINCIPLES OF PAIN CONTROL

Try to define the type and site of pain

Careful history-taking and examination, occasionally supplemented by investigations, will usually demonstrate pain of one or more of the following types:-

1. Bone pain, usually described as a dull, deep ache in the whole length of a bone with a localized area of greater intensity, often over the site of metastases in the case of cancer.
2. Nerve root compression, clearly localized to anatomical dermatomes. Here the history is all important. For example, if the patient has minimal pain when lying but it worsens in the dorsal lumbar spine sitting and is unbearable on standing, radiating down (e.g.) L1, it can safely be assumed there is compression of L1. This is confirmed by the history of it being exacerbated by coughing, sneezing or straining. Examination may be unrewarding.
3. Colic — no different in chronic conditions than in acute ones, coming on suddenly, short-lived but intense, and producing a sense of collapse.
4. Headache, nearly always due to either raised intracranial pressure from a space-occupying lesion, or bone metastases in the cranium, again suspected from the history. That due to intracranial pressure is described as a 'vice around the head', worse on wakening and often absent from mid-morning onwards. When due to metastases, there is often a localized area of pain and tenderness on gentle palpation or percussion.
5. Skin hyperaesthesia is well recognized by nurses who care for

stroke patients but is sometimes found in oat cell bronchogenic carcinoma, melanomatosis, and the reticuloses. Light touch is unpleasant, bed clothes too heavy, but firm handling much preferred.

6. Visceral pain is experienced when a viscus expands and stretches its sensitive capsule. In the case of the liver this is first felt under the lower right ribs then as the hepatomegaly advances, in the right hypochondrium. By this time the patient usually prefers to lie on the right side, objects to lying on his back, and cannot bear to lie for long either flat or bolt upright because the liver-edge is then pressed against the abdominal wall or pelvic bone.

   A cause of acute-on-chronic pain in such patients is the sudden pain felt in the enlarged liver when bleeding occurs in a secondary deposit.

7. Joint pain, no different from any of the arthridities. It is easy to forget that a terminal illness does not cure long-standing arthritis though it may divert the patient's attention from it. When the newer pain of his cancer is relieved he again becomes aware of the hip or fingers which have troubled him for so long.

8. Muscular pain felt in affected muscles when put under strain for any reason, even the gentle handling by a nurse.

The reason for attempting to define pain in this way is that every effort may be made to:

Try to treat each pain specifically

Admittedly this is not always possible but at least it can be attempted. Raised intracranial pressure may be reduced by dexamethasone, bone pain by a prostaglandin biosynthetase inhibitor, hyperaesthesia by a peripheral-acting analgesic, nerve root compression by steroids or nerve blocks and so forth.

Anticipate pain breakthrough

By definition chronic pain keeps on recurring. There is therefore, with only one exception, no place for PRN prescribing which places a burdensome responsibility on the patient, courageously to bear the pain as long as possible without resorting to analgesics. Doing this may give him the impression that it is either dangerous to take his drug regularly or that he is expected to suffer a little. It is analogous to asking a diabetic to take his insulin only if he finds himself going into a diabetic coma! Dying patients have enough to suffer without having to earn their analgesia.

The secret is to prescribe analgesics at intervals determined by their period of efficacy in chronic pain to prevent pain breakthrough.

Review the regime frequently and regularly

It is sometimes not appreciated how quickly a terminally ill patient's condition changes. Today's pain-free patient may tomorrow have a new pain which requires a different drug.

Remember that you are treating 'total pain'

The dying patient is not a malignant secondary deposit! He is someone with profound and often complex emotional needs and problems, a social and a domestic life, and a spiritual dimension to his being. Each affects his attitude to pain, his threshold for pain, and his response not only to his drugs but everything else which is happening to him. No one is better qualified or placed to care for the 'whole' man and his 'total' pain than the family doctor.

SPECIFIC PAINS:

As stated, every effort should be made to prescribe specifically.

Bone pain

The first line of treatment for a malignant deposit should be palliative radiotherapy, remembering that at least three to four weeks may elapse before benefit is felt. Such irradiation is remarkably non-upsetting, in contrast to the side effects of irradiation of such sensitive tissues as the gastrointestinal tract and bladder. It is a professional kindness to send a patient even some distance to the nearest centre for radiation oncology rather than wait until the pain is uncontrollable with analgesic drugs. It must also be remembered that a considerable amount of bone destruction has to have occurred before it will be demonstrated on straight X-ray films. The suspicion of bone metastases should be the signal for referral, possible bone scan and radiotherapy. Most patients will need full-dose prostaglandin biosynthetase inhibitors, acting as they do on the PGE_2 released by bone deposits. Which one is employed will be dictated by the patient's history of dyspepsia, ability to swallow tablets and comply with instructions.

Certainly until the irradiation has taken effect, most will need strong analgesics of the opiate family. The doctor will know when to reduce the dose, or even stop the drug, when the side effects such as sedation become evident, showing that the pain has been reduced by irradiation. It cannot be stated strongly enough that *pain is the physiological antagonist to the opiates.* So long as he has pain there are few dangers in using these drugs. When pain has been brought under control, by radiotherapy or nerve blocks, the dose may need to be brought down.

Nerve root compression

When pain is confined to two or three adjacent dermatomes, it is an indication for considering the place of nerve blocks and appropriate referral be made at once to the nearest Pain Relief Clinic or hospice.

The following broad guidelines may be useful here:
1. *intercostal blocks* — for unilateral pain in the dermatomes of the thoracic area, e.g. for pain localized to a breast carcinoma, myeloma, mesothelioma or other chest wall deposits, or lesions of the upper abdominal wall
2. *intrathecal/epidural blocks* — for similar lesions (when more prolonged effect is called for) and for unilateral pain in dermatomes D2 to L2
3. *coeliac plexus block* — for the pain of pancreatic carcinoma and some pains in the perineum and lower one-third rectum
4. *caudal blocks* — for pain in S4 and S5 particularly in patients with a colostomy and catheter when a neurolytic agent can be expected to impair bowel and bladder sphincter control.

The chemical most commonly used is phenol in glycerine and benefit can be expected to last for eight to twelve weeks, after which, should pain recur, the procedure can often be repeated.

If for some reason a nerve block is not indicated, benefit may follow the prescription of a steroid (dexamethasone 4 mg daily) to reduce perineural oedema.

Usually a strong analgesic is also required but frequently this pain is helped by the combination of a low-dose central-acting analgesic (e.g. an opiate or dextropropoxyphene) and a peripheral actor such a salicylate.

Raised intracranial pressure

Both the headache and vomiting may be relieved by dexamethasone, initially 16 mg daily, reduced as speedily as possible to a maintenance dose of 6 – 8 mg daily. Seldom do the opiates by themselves achieve benefit in this condition.

It must be remembered that steroids such as dexamethasone are, in fact, life-support systems—easy to start, difficult to stop. The initial benefit may be dramatic only to be followed by a prolongation of life associated with added strain on the family and all the adverse effects of the drugs, not least of which are Cushing's syndrome and proximal myopathy.

Visceral pain

Though strong analgesics are almost always required, benefit may occasionally follow the use of high-dose steroids, either orally or by injection, for a week.

NON-SPECIFIC ANALGESIA

The rule is to start with low-potency analgesics and build up to the maximum recommended, tolerated dose. When this is achieved and pain then breaks through, one moves to the medium-potency group and finally the stronger group which includes all the commonly used narcotics. There is no indication for moving backwards and forwards from one group to another.

Some examples may be useful here. For a while the pain may be relieved with paracetamol 1 g 4-hourly. When this proves inadequate, the drug is stopped and replaced with (e.g.) dipipanone starting with 10 mg 6-hourly, increased as required to 20 mg 6-hourly. When the disease has progressed sufficiently to merit something stronger, the doctor remembers that dipipanone 10 mg equals oral morphine 5 mg (Table 1) and therefore his patient is taking the equivalent of 40 mg of morphine daily. To control the pain he will need 60 mg oral morphine each day, taken as either morphine solution 10 mg every 4 hours *or* MST 30 mg every 12 hours, depending on how rapidly the condition is developing.

Table 1 Narcotic equivalents

Oral dipipanone	10 mg	
Oral papaveretum	10 mg	} Oral morphine 5 mg
Oral levorphanol	1.5 mg	

USE OF OPIATES

Contrary to what was long held to be the case, there are minimal dangers of respiratory depression with morphine and diamorphine given regularly for terminal cancer pain. Neither need the doctor fear that they will be used to commit suicide, or that nausea or vomiting will persist beyond the first four days or so of their use, nor that the patient will experience anything worse than inactivity drowsiness. The question of addiction is a *non-issue* in such patients and opiate tolerance is seldom, if ever, a problem — increase in dose almost always being associated with disease progression rather than true pharmacological tolerance.

There is no doubt whatsoever that opiates are often withheld from dying patients for quite unscientific, unjustified reasons. They will be found indispensable in at least 60% of those dying from terminal cancer. The earlier they are prescribed the greater the likelihood that the dose may eventually be reduced.

For oral administration, the drug of choice is morphine. It is made up in tap water or chloroform water, preferably in a 10 ml dose, and must be given *4-hourly round the clock*. Only when the dose requirement has been established can the patient be given a double dose at 10 p.m. and omit the 2 a.m. dose.

When the morphine requirement has already been defined from the intake of the solution *or* when analgesic requirements are very slowly increasing in a slowly advancing cancer, the morphine may be given as MST 12-hourly. However, it must be remembered that this controlled release preparation takes approximately four hours to achieve satisfactory plasma levels. It cannot be employed for 'breakthrough' pain and need *never* be given more frequently than 8-hourly.

MORPHINE OR DIAMORPHINE?

Contrary to long-held beliefs, there is nothing to choose between these opiates provided certain principles are remembered (Table 2):
1. *Oral* diamorphine is 1.5 times as potent as *oral* morphine, i.e. diamorphine 10 mg = morphine 15 mg.

Table 2 Morphine equivalents

Oral diamorphine	5 mg =	Oral morphine 7.5 mg [1:1.5]
Oral methadone	5 mg =	Oral morphine 7.5 mg [1:1.5]
Oral phenazocine	5 mg =	Oral morphine 25 mg [1:5]
Inj. diamorphine	5 mg =	Oral morphine 15 mg [1:3]

2. *Subcutaneous* diamorphine is 3 times as potent as *oral* morphine, i.e. s.c. diamorphine 10 mg = *oral* morphine 30 mg.
3. Morphine is the preferable drug for oral solution because it can so easily be titrated to the patient's needs.
4. Diamorphine should be the opiate employed for injection because of its remarkably high solubility and therefore small volume required for injection.
5. Diamorphine solution is converted into morphine within a few weeks, hence unused diamorphine solution should not be stored either in the patient's home or doctor's surgery.

Both drugs constipate and a prescription of an adjuvant laxative is therefore mandatory.

ALTERNATIVE ROUTES FOR NARCOTIC ADMINISTRATION (Tables 3 and 4)

As explained, the doctor will usually commence with oral morphine solution until the dose requirement is ascertained. If the pain is rapidly increasing, and therefore the requirement of morphine also rising in parallel, he will persist with this solution. If the requirement is static, he will probably consider MST, giving the 24 hours requirement in three equal doses every 8 hours.

Table 3 Duration of effectiveness: oral narcotics

Dextromoramide	2 hours
Pethidine	3 hours
Morphine	
Diamorphine	4 hours
Papaveretum	
Dipipanane	
Phenazocine	6 hours
Levorphanol	
Methadone	8 hours
Buprenorphine	
Morphine sustained	10–12 hours
Release (MST)	

Table 4 Duration of effectiveness: injected narcotics

Dextromoramide	1–1½ hours
Pethidine	2 hours
Morphine	
Diamorphine	3–4 hours
Phenazocine	6 hours
Methadone	6–8 hours

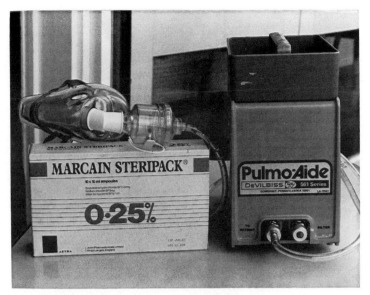

Figure 1 Marcain nebuliser

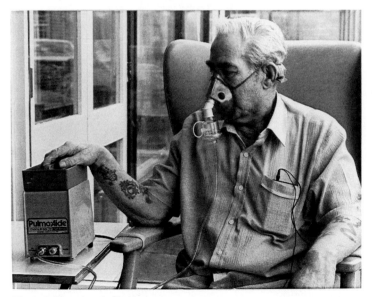

Figure 2 Marcain nebuliser in use

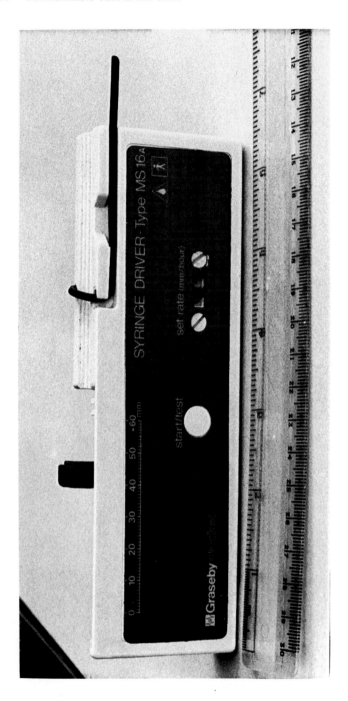

Figure 3 Syringe driver

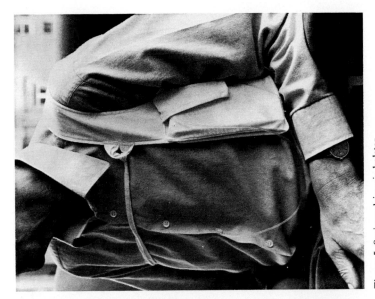

Figure 5 Syringe driver in holster

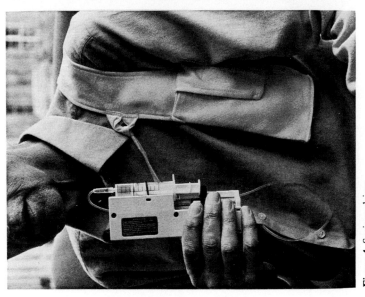

Figure 4 Syringe driver

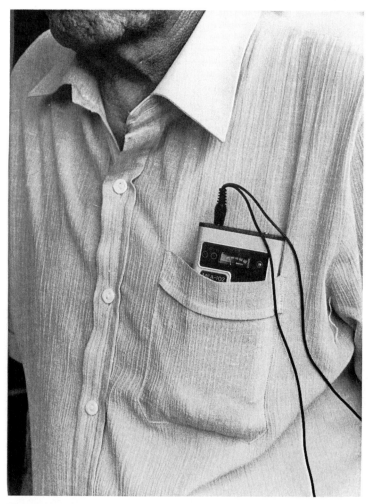

Figure 6 Transcutaneous electric nerve stimulator (TENS)

Alternative routes of administration will have to be considered when:
1. persistent vomiting is a problem;
2. there is doubt that the drug is being absorbed;
3. the patient cannot tolerate the taste of the solution or is unable or unwilling to swallow tablets.

The choice will then be between the following.

A change to 4-hourly subcutaneous diamorphine

The total intake of morphine in the previous 24 hours is divided by 3 and then 1/6th of that administered 4-hourly. For example, a patient finding difficulty taking oral morphine 30 mg every 4 hours is receiving 180 mg in 24 hours, equivalent to 60 mg of subcutaneous diamorphine. A 4-hourly injection would be 10 mg.

A less laborious way of calculation is obviously to give one-third of the oral morphine dose every 4 hours as diamorphine injection.

A change to morphine suppositories

Though no exact analgesic equivalent can be given, rectal administration is not quite as predictable as the oral. It is prudent to regard the suppository as approximately two-thirds of the oral.

Another example may assist here. A patient on oral morphine 20 mg every 4 hours will require not less than morphine suppository 30 mg every 6 hours, possibly every 4 hours.

A change to diamorphine by syringe-driver (Table 5)

These miniature, pocket-sized, battery-operated pumps have revolutionalized domiciliary terminal care in recent years but there is a danger that they are being used more often than is really necessary and sometimes for convenience rather than good scientific reasons. Nevertheless they must be regarded as an essential piece of equipment in large practices and Health Centres where there is often likely to be at least one patient posing a problem of pain control with advanced cancer. They can enable a patient to be attended by a nurse (at least for his analgesic control) once daily whereas if he were on 4-hourly injections, it might well prove inpracticable for the busy community nursing service to cope with such as pattern of visiting. The 10 ml syringe is loaded with a 24-hour requirement of diamorphine dissolved in water for injection

Table 5 Using a syringe driver

1. Insert a battery, press starter button and check that the light is flashing.
2. Dissolve 24-hour requirement of diamorphine in 10 ml 'water for injection' using a standard 10 ml disposable syringe.
3. Affix butterfly needle on the longest available polythene lead, to syringe and expel solution to needle tip.
4. Secure syringe to syringe driver and fasten firmly.
5. Insert needle subcutaneously in anterior abdominal wall, anterior axillary fold or over deltoid insertion.
6. Keep needle in place with 'micropore', or other non-allergenic, transparent seal.
7. Set syringe driver at '2' for infusion over 24 hours and house it in plastic cover provided.
8. Place syringe driver in holster, pocket or under the pillow.
9. Check the rate of infusion every 6 or 12 hours until it is assured pump is infusing satisfactorily.
10. Resite needle every 4 or 5 days (unless an inflammatory reaction appears).
11. Replace needle and giving set every 14 days.

and secured to the syringe-driver. To it, is affixed a butterfly needle on a polythene line, the needle inserted *subcutaneously* (not i.v.) in the anterior abdominal wall, anterior axillary line, or over the insertion of deltoid, held in place with Steri-strips, Micropore or Opsite. The driver is set at the arbitrary figure of '2' for 24-hour infusion, and the pump started by inserting the battery. A freshly loaded syringe is prepared and affixed by the nurse at approximately the same time each day. It should be noted that the needle can be left *in situ* for, on average, four days and then re-used in a different site. A new needle and giving set is needed every fourteen days.

Experience has shown that many adjuvants can be added to the diamorphine solution including haloperidol, promazine, cyclizine, chlorpromazine, methotrimeprazine, prochlorperazine and hyoscine. Frusemide certainly cannot be added and possibly not dexamethasone.

The difficulties which may be encountered include:

1. The patient may prefer regular injections because in that way he will feel he is getting more attention. Others may, initially, be put off by the 'technology'.
2. Sterile inflammatory reactions may develop at the injection site, particularly with high-dose diamorphine. This merely calls for more frequent change of site. It is impossible to quote a dose when this may be expected but in Hospice experience it is relatively common with 500 mg or more of diamorphine. It is *not* usually an indication for discontinuing this route of administration.

3. The pump may run in too fast (in which case the rate is slowed down) or too slowly when for days or weeks it has been satisfactory. This requires a new battery!
4. The cachectic patient has little subcutaneous tissue left and the solution merely pools under the skin. Where this happens there is no alternative to regular s.c. injections unless the dose is so small that an equivalent can be given by morphine suppository.
5. In a few areas there remains some uncertainty about community nurses making up the diamorphine solution and loading the syringe-driver apparently because, through ignorance, a higher authority believes it is being given intravenously.

A change to another narcotic other than an opiate

There are no better analgesics than the opiates and all alternatives, numerous as they are, have several disadvantages.

Methadone

This may be given as tablet, injection (s.c., i.m., or by syringe-driver) or elixir. (It should be noted that the proprietary preparation Physeptone Linctus only contains 2 mg/5 ml and is therefore primarily a cough suppressant.) When an analgesic strength is called for, the appropriate dose can be prescribed and made up specially by the pharmacist.

However, it has to be remembered that methadone is a marked respiratory depressant, has a long half-life, and a very unpredictable analgesic effect. It is 1.5 times as potent as oral morphine (i.e. the same as diamorphine) but tolerance develops rapidly.

It is essential for the doctor to plan his home visiting carefully for any patient whom he has changed to methadone, ensuring that he revisits in 36 hours because of the delayed effect.

Again, an example may help. A patient requiring to be changed from oral morphine 5 mg every 4 hours (30 mg in 24 hours) would initially need 5 mg every 8 hours but within days, probably, 5 mg every 6 hours (20 mg in 24 hours).

Buprenorphine

The convenience of this preparation has to be admitted. It can slowly be increased to cope with the increasing pain, starting with one tablet (0.2 mg) every 12 hours, and eventually giving 0.4 mg every 4 hours. There are however major limitations. There is an analgesic ceiling (0.4 mg 4-hourly) beyond which there will be no increased benefit. The sublingual tablet may be poorly absorbed in the mouth of a patient either dehydrated or suffering a dry mouth. More important is the fact that it is a partial antagonist making it difficult, though not impossible, to change to a pure agonist, such as morphine or diamorphine. Some would suggest an increased dose equivalent of the agonist for the first 12 hours after stopping the buprenorphine and commencing the morphine. The approximate analgesic equivalent is 60:1, buprenorphine to morphine, e.g. a patient on buprenorphine 0.4 mg 12-hourly would need 48 mg in 24 hours of oral morphine, or to make it easier and recognize that a stronger dose is needed for the increasing pain, 60 mg given as 10 mg oral morphine solution every 4 hours.

What then are the indications for buprenorphine in domiciliary terminal care?

1. An easily administered analgesic for the patient whose pain is too severe for a low-strength analgesic (aspirin, codeine, mefenamic acid, dextropropoxyphene etc.), yet not severe enough to merit an opiate.
2. For the patient whose pain is increasing very slowly, necessitating infrequent increases in analgesia, probably over many weeks or months. It is not the right drug for the patient whose analgesic requirements are changing every few days, nor for the patient expected to need an opiate within a short time. Such a patient should be started on the opiate from the outset rather than on buprenorphine.
3. The patient who cannot swallow tablets or, for any reason, cannot or will not take oral morphine solution.

In the opinion of the author, buprenorphine is a useful drug in general practice for mild to severe pain but rarely the drug of choice for the pain experienced by the dying cancer patient.

Dextramoramide

This drug, marketed as Palfium, comes in 5 mg and 10 mg tablets which can be taken sublingually (avoiding first-pass metabolism) or may be swallowed or given by suppository. It can be expected to be effective within 10 to 15 minutes sublingually but remain effective for little more than two hours. It has to be admitted that, useful as it is, remarkably little documentary evidence is available on its use and period of efficacy in terminal care.

It is three times as potent as oral morphine (dextramoramide 5 mg = oral morphine 15 mg) but suffers from rapid development of tolerance and an analgesic ceiling. It should *never* be given on a regular basis.

The indications for its use are:

1. For 'breakthrough' pain in the patient on 4-hourly morphine who very occasionally experiences pain before the next dose is due.
2. For analgesia during painful procedures, such as extensive prolonged dressings and bladder lavage. The doctor who assists his community nurse colleague by prescribing sublingual dextramoramide for her to perform such a task will not only help his patient but win the respect of the nurse.
3. For the patient who has occasional attacks of particularly severe pain which require immediate analgesia before the doctor can reach the house. The causes of such pain might be haemorrhage in a hepatic secondary deposit, a pathological fractured rib in a patient with myelomatosis and the patient who develops painful clot retention with carcinoma of bladder.

Dextromoramide is a valuable drug not sufficiently used in domiciliary terminal care but is *not* a substitute for the opiates.

Phenazocine

Marketed as a 5 mg scored tablet (Narphen), this analgesic has five times the potency of oral morphine (i.e. phenazocine 5 mg = oral morphine 25 mg) and can be swallowed or sucked sublingually. Like the opiates it is antagonized by naloxone (Narcan).

Sadly, it too has disadvantages. It is respiratory depressant, is unpredictable in its side effects—sometimes being very sedative and in other patients having no sedative properties whatsoever. In some it is very nauseating but exceptionally well tolerated in others. Some older patients may experience most distressing hallucinations.

It is, however, less constipating than the opiates, need only be administered 6-hourly (provided the dose is slowly built up) and can, on occasions, be a useful substitute for morphine. Generally, however, the patient who cannot tolerate morphine is also intolerant of phenazocine.

Other drugs

There are other drugs which should be mentioned only to be dismissed.

Pethidine has almost no place in terminal care. It is a weak narcotic, very much less potent than morphine in patients with advanced carcinoma, tends to be nauseating, develops tolerance rapidly and is probably effective by mouth for no longer than three hours, and one hour by injection. Its use as an antispasmodic is rarely called for in terminal care because colic is so unusual even in patients with sub-acute obstruction.

Pentazocine (Fortral) is too weak to be of use in anything other than mild pain, and too hallucinogenic for such patients as we are discussing.

Nefopam (Acupan) is a unique drug whose mode and site of action are ill-understood. It may have a place in the management of mild pain but has been shown to be epileptogenic.

Dipipanone (Diconal) is a popular drug, sadly combined quite unnecessarily with cyclizine, and has an analgesic ratio with oral morphine of 2:1 (i.e. dipipanone 10 mg = oral morphine 5 mg) making conversion easy. Its usefulness in terminal care is limited by its maximum recommended dose of 20 mg (2 tablets) 6-hourly, equivalent to only 40 mg oral morphine in 24 hours.

In summary, there are no better analgesics in terminal care than opiates. Skilfully used they are capable of controlling the pain of almost all dying patients. There should only be rare occasions in a doctor's professional lifetime when he will need to take a patient off them, usually for uncontrollable confusion which it will always be difficult to attribute to these drugs to the exclusion of any other cause.

Extremely valuable as the opiates are, their benefits can often be enhanced (though not strictly potentiated) by the equally skilled use of adjuvants.

ADJUVANT DRUGS FOR ANALGESIA

In addition to the prostaglandin biosynthetase inhibitors (NSAIDs) already referred to for the pain of bone secondaries, the most commonly used drugs are as follows:

Phenothiazines

The principal ones are chlorpromazine, prochlorperazine, methotrimeprazine, and pericyazine (though not strictly a phenothiazine). They all have sedative potential with methotrimeprazine the most sedative. All are, in varying degree, anti-emetic and all are capable of producing Parkinsonian features though pericyazine is less likely than the others to do so.

Useful indications in domiciliary terminal care include:

1. Chlorpromazine suppositories at night, remembering that by this route the 100 mg suppository is approximately equivalent to 50 mg orally.
2. Methotrimeprazine (tablet Veractil or injection Nozinam) as a sedative with a unique analgesic property in its own right although tolerance appears to develop and injections may have to be given 4-hourly (or by syringe-driver) with the effect wearing off suddenly. Within minutes the deeply asleep patient may be sitting up, alert or even agitated.
3. Pericyazine for the aggressive, agitated patient with a personality problem, either pre-existent or resulting from intracerebral pathology.

Benzodiazepines

In the opinion of the author, these tranquillizers are often preferable to the phenothiazines because the patient feels less 'vague' and 'detached' and their anxiolytic effect (as opposed to the sedative effect) is more apparent.

1. Lorazepam (orally or sublingually) is useful for panic attacks which the doctor or nurse may recognize as such rather than breakthrough pain but which the patient will more usually describe as pain, often in very graphic detail if he or she has a hysterical personality. Some patients will settle to sleep more rapidly with this drug than with a related benzodiazepine such as temazepam.
2. Diazepam — once daily because of its long half-life is valuable to the patient whose fear or terror (sometimes impossible to define or unravel) is creating muscle tension, serving only to aggravate the pain.

In terminal care, one occasionally comes across a patient whose 'pain' seems impossible to control or define. The question eventually changes from 'What exactly is causing the pain and why is it not responding?' to 'How much of the so-called pain is really a cry from the heart which no opiate will help?' Even after hours of listening and the skilled attention of each member of the primary care team no progress has been made. The solution may lie in tranquillizing that patient with diazepam, initially giving it by mouth or suppository twice daily, then maintaining on a nightly dose. There appears to be a cross tolerance with the opiates which is so far unexplained, calling for a higher dose for diazepam in patients already on high-dose opiates.

Histamine antagonists

Cimetidine in the same dose as for peptic ulcer, or ranitidine when there is liver disfunction, are useful adjuvants for the pain and other symptoms of gastric, oesophageal or stoma carcinomata.

The pain of post-radiation oesophagitis may be helped by simple analgesics or, occasionally required, carbenoxolone in the form of Biogastrone sucked four times daily.

Tricyclic antidepressants

Amitriptyline in the dose of 75 mg each night will be found helpful for some dysaesthetic pain and, so some believe, as an adjuvant in other difficult to control pains mediated via the spinal-thalamic pathways.

Though undoubtedly the incidence of 'endogenous' depression is no higher in the dying than in the general population and most of the depression encountered in the terminally ill reflects poorly managed symptoms or unexpressed sadness and fear, nevertheless a therapeutic trial of an antidepressant is sometimes justified when pain is providing difficult to control.

Steroids

Their uses are many in terminal care but undoubtedly they are useful for nerve entrapment pain by reducing the perineural oedema. An average dose might be dexamethasone 4 mg each morning or prednisolone 10 mg tid.

Last, but by no means least, is the alleviation of BOREDOM — one of the greatest challenges of terminal care whether at home or in hospital or hospice. There is ample evidence that the pain threshold is raised when the cerebrum is bombarded with many visual, auditory, and other sensory impulses, whether they come from a well-planned environment, a well-positioned bed by a window, TV programmes, reading matter, skilled visitors, or even a busy ward. In the same way we all know that a patient whose mind is usefully occupied or who is enabled to feel useful to others, both experiences and reports less pain than the bored patient.

It is probably one of the supreme tests of a doctor's or nurse's skills to help a dying patient not only to have less pain but to feel that what life he has left is still a useful and appreciated one.

The control of pain is a challenge to the primary care team. It requires consummate skills in prescribing appropriate drugs, manipulating the environment, alleviating fears and building up a relationship of trust. It can almost as easily be achieved at home as in the best hospice. It requires no gimmicks, no sophisticated equipment — only professionals who are prepared to make the necessary effort.

2

Symptom control

In acute medical conditions each symptom has a diagnostic significance which, taken with a careful examination and the necessary
investigations, should lead to a diagnosis and appropriate treatment
for the *disease* and not the symptom. Patients understand this
and are usually eager to report most symptoms in some detail in the
hope that this will assist the clinician to help or cure them.

In chronic conditions, and especially in far-advanced and terminal illness, symptoms have less diagnostic value to the clinician
but for the patient are a reminder of worsening suffering and
increasing threat to his life, his independence, and his dignity. No
more than 50% of these distressing symptoms are usually reported
to his attendant, lest they are thought too trivial. The sense of
professional disappointment at being unable to cure or control the
disease can display itself to the patient in less interest being shown
in any symptom which has no apparent diagnostic value, or is
difficult to alleviate. The result is a vicious circle of more suffering
endured in silence, often in fear, each new experience depressing
the patient further and isolating him from family and professional
attendants.

The terminally ill fear the unknown more than the known,
professional disinterest more than professional ineptitude, the process of dying rather than death itself. They seldom, if ever, expect
every distress to be removed. They do, however, ask that interest
be shown in their distress, that its significance be explained, and
the opportunity be made available for them to speak of *anything*
which, at any time, seems importance to them. The more ill the
patient, the more relevant each symptom becomes in relation to his
family rather than to himself. For example, he may have no
personal discomfort with his halitosis yet may become isolated from
his wife because of it. Such suffering is no less important to him
and merits no less attention from his attendants.

The fact that the patient is known to have a fatal illness in no way lessens the need for accurate history taking, examination and appropriate investigations. The only difference, and one usually well recognized by the patient, is that *treatment is directed at alleviation of symptoms rather than eradication of a disease.*

Obvious rules apply to such treatment:

1. It must be simple, readily understood by the patient (and attendants), tailored to his changing needs and his ability to comply with instructions.
2. It must be reviewed regularly and frequently, as carefully as in acute conditions.
3. It must be explained to the patient and all his attendants after honest explanations of the significance of each symptom.
4. It must not, in any way, worsen his suffering or increase his disability or fear.

By this stage of an illness, *the patient is more concerned with his distress than his diagnosis.*

IT CANNOT BE STATED STRONGLY ENOUGH THAT BY THE TIME A PATIENT ENTERS THE LAST MONTHS OF HIS LIFE WITH A CHRONIC PROGRESSIVE ILLNESS, PARTICULARLY MALIGNANT DISEASE, WHETHER HE ADMITS IT TO ALL AND SUNDRY OR NOT, HE IS USUALLY AWARE OF THE DIAGNOSIS AND ITS FATAL OUTCOME.

ANOREXIA (see Chapter 4)

Causes

1. Oral thrush (present in 75% of patients)
2. Chronic constipation
3. Uninteresting, unimaginative food
4. Too large helpings, or food offered only at standard meal times
5. Odours in environment
6. Nausea and vomiting
7. Excessive medication and/or dry mouth (itself often drug-induced)
8. Depressive state
9. Metabolic — hypercalcaemia, uraemia.

Management

1. Try to remove the offending cause.

2. The nearer the patient is to death the colder does he prefer all drinks, and the less does he want sweet things.
3. Tempt the patient with minute helpings on the smallest plate available.
4. Offer attractively served food at frequent intervals unrelated to standard meal times. (Many patients will prefer to eat porridge at night and to eat ice cream or yogurt in the morning. Breakfast is nearly always appreciated even in patients not eating in the remaining 24 hours.)
5. Offer a small alcoholic drink of his choice as an aperitif.
6. Be reluctant to offer 'invalid' food no matter how nutritious, but ever ready to permit and encourage any bizarre fancies the patient may have even if it is 'Chinese carry-out', kippers during the night, lager at breakfast, stout with added sugar.
7. Dexamethasone 2 mg each morning, unless strongly contraindicated. *This is the only 'tonic' recognized as having any efficacy in appetite stimulation.*

ANTIBIOTICS IN TERMINAL CARE

Antibiotics should only be used in terminal care
1. When there are good reasons for thinking that the patient's present symptoms are due to, or aggravated by, an easily treatable infection — for example in chest or bladder.
2. When the treatment is not going to be more unpleasant for the patient than the symptoms themselves.

They should not be used indiscriminately for patients with lung cancer suffering increasing cough and breathlessness but only where infection is evident and treatable.

Similarly, urinary symptoms might well be due to local invasion of the bladder by pelvic tumour or due to the presence of accumulating ascites.

The side effects of some antibiotics — oral thrush, nausea, diarrhoea, and secondary infection by resistant organisms — may be much more unpleasant and difficult to treat than the original infection.

ANXIETY

It is impossible to imagine any dying patient who will not show some features of anxiety if he has poorly controlled pain, recurrent vomiting, disabling dyspnoea even at rest, bleeding from any site, dysphagia or any other major distress.

Even patients with no personality disorder and no past history of anxiety neurosis will be anxious to a 'pathological degree' if

1. Pain or any other distress is not taken seriously by professional attendants and given energetic treatment.
2. The significance to the patient of each new distress is not explored and explained in simple, honest terms, remembering that the significance to the patient may be quite different from that to the professional. Their palpitations may be thought of as 'the cancer reaching the heart', sweating as a sign of tuberculosis, while oedema is 'renal failure', poor visual acuity as incipient blindness etc.
3. Different professional attendants, nurses and doctors, give different and apparently conflicting explanations, prognosis and advice.

Management

1. No anxiolytic is as effective as time spent sharing a patient's problem and ensuring he is as fully in the picture about his illness and its features as his intelligence, education and state of health will permit. This requires not so much *quantity* of time spent with a patient as *quality* of time. The dying are usually acutely aware of how little time is left to them and how busy are their professional attendants and ask only that these attendants take them and their troubles seriously. A few minutes of serious concentrated attention are more valuable to them than half an hour of light superficial conversation when something is troubling them.
2. The best 'anxiolytics' are those which relieve the distressing symptoms, whether appropriate analgesics for pain, steroids for anorexia, laxatives for constipation or anti-emetics for vomiting.
3. When all else has been tried only then should the true anxiolytics be prescribed, preferably early morning and late at night when anxiety and pain are usually most evident and alarming, or at night only when a long half-life benzodiazepine is used.
4. When tablets cannot be swallowed it is worth remembering that lorazepam can be sucked sublingually, or diazepam be given as suppositories (2, 5, 10 mg).
5. Panic attacks are best treated by the presence of a reassuring attendant, sublingual lorazepam 0.5–1 mg, or diazepam rectal

solution 10–20 mg. The latter is effective within ten to fifteen minutes and lasts no longer than three hours. It is sometimes forgotten that intramuscular diazepam takes longer to become effective than oral or rectal solution, has a long half-life, tends to accumulate, and is capable of producing respiratory depression.

6. When pain is a feature of the condition, and of sufficient degree to merit consideration of an opiate, it should be remembered that morphine and diamorphine remain both the best analgesics *and* anxiolytics.

BLOOD TRANSFUSION

Chronic anaemia is common in the terminal stages of advanced cancer. Symptoms and signs associated with anaemia include:

dyspnoea	pallor
faintness	angina
palpitations	drowsiness
lethargy	confusion

but they are seldom significant unless the haemoglobin is below 8 g/dl. The decision whether or not to tranfuse is made more difficult by the fact that:

1. many of these features are also those of advanced cancer;
2. previous tranfusions may have produced a placebo effect influencing the patient's view on its benefit.

Indications for transfusion

1. Symptoms thought to be *directly* due to the anaemia (and not the underlying cancer) where the patient's activity is limited by the anaemia and where the haemoglobin is less than 8 g/dl.
2. Unequivocal evidence of benefit from a previous transfusion.

A blood transfusion should not be given merely to treat a low haemoglobin, or in the hope that it will make the patient feel better or to help the doctor feel he is 'doing something'.

CONFUSION

Confusion is a common and distressing problem. Remember that the patient who is very deaf or very anxious might not be confused at all in spite of what other colleagues might say.

Causes of confusion (not an exhaustive list)

1. *Uncontrolled pain*, unrecognized discomfort due to urinary retention or severe constipation.
2. *Changes in the environment*, leaving home, transfer from one ward to another.
3. *Metabolic disturbance*, septicaemia, uraemia, hypercalcaemia, hyponatraemia, hypoxia.
4. *Cerebral metastases.*
5. *Cerebral vascular disease.*
6. *Drug-induced*, for example psychotropic drugs, barbiturates and cimetidine.
7. *Drug withdrawal* may also precipitate confusion, for example, alcohol, benzodiazepines, barbiturates, opiates.

Management of confusion

1. Alleviate any identifiable cause if possible and if appropriate.
2. Confident handling by a limited number of staff and with relative always close at hand. A single room always well lit will help.
3. Sedation (for both the patient, the relatives' and the staff's sake).
   a. Diazepam 5–10 ml orally or by suppository (if the confusion is severe then the use of an intravenous preparation such as Diazemuls might be indicated).
   b. Chlorpromazine 25–50 mg tds orally or intramuscularly.
   c. Methotrimeprazine (a more sedative phenothiazine) 25–50 mg 4–8 hourly.
   d. Haloperidol is valuable if there are associated hallucinations and paranoia (1.5–5 mg orally or intramuscularly tds).
   e. Pericyazine 5–10 mg tds particularly where the confusion is associated with aggressive behaviour or a personality change.

CONSTIPATION

Of patients seen by terminal care teams in hospitals and the community 75–80% are found to be very constipated. Unimportant as the condition is considered by many doctors it is the commonest cause of vomiting in the terminally ill, a common cause of unnecessary abdominal discomfort and anorexia, and a source of considerable anxiety to many patients, particularly the elderly, who see it as further evidence of breakdown in their body's basic functions. Professional reassurance that it is not serious or life-threatening does not help. It is usually possible both to prevent it and correct it.

Causes

1. Impaired fluid intake or excessive loss through vomiting, tachypnoea, or sweating.
2. A small food intake of predominantly low roughage, high milk-content diet ('invalid foods').
3. Relative immobility.
4. Drug-induced (opiates, tricyclic antidepressants, phenothiazine tranquillizers, anticholinergic drugs, cough sedatives etc.).

Management

The normal regime of encouraging a diet of bran, fibre, fruit and fluids is not usually appropriate in a patient seldom able to take them. Even bran added to porridge and soup is seldom acceptable. Laxatives are required and the patient encouraged to maintain a reasonable fluid intake.

Examination

It cannot be stressed strongly enough that rectal examinations must be carried out on all patients.

1. When the rectum is found to be filled with hard faecal masses do NOT give any faecal expander which will only convert a small hard mass into a large soft one, impossible to expel. Give an arachis oil enema at night on two successive nights, followed by two bisacodyl suppositories or a phosphate enema in the morning.
2. When the rectum is empty but ballooned, signifying faecal impaction around the rectosigmoid junction, do *not* give a faecal expander alone without a peristaltic stimulant, nor use suppositories. The only effective treatment will be lactulose accompanied by senna tablets or bisacodyl tablets with daily rectal examinations to ensure that the mass is not collecting in the lower rectum. When it does, the patient requires phosphate enemata.
3. When the rectum is empty and collapsed, there is no faecal

impaction and oral faecal expanders/peristaltic stimulants will be effective.

Maintenance regime

1. When opiates are used the strongest laxative will always be required on a regular basis, e.g. lactulose reducing from 20 ml tid to 10–20 ml bd. It is essential to start with the higher dose, gradually reducing over the following week.
2. With lactulose a peristaltic stimulant is often required. There is little to choose between them, the choice usually depending on patient compliance and acceptance.

COUGH

Whilst dyspnoea and breathlessness are often encountered in terminal care, cough is less common than might be expected except in lung cancer. This is fortunate because, unless the underlying cause can be removed, there are few truly effective measures for it.

Causes

1. Bronchial obstruction from a primary tumour or mediastinal mass, most commonly enlarged mediastinal glands.
2. Secondary bronchial infection, pneumonia or an abscess in necrotic tumour.
3. Left ventricular failure with characteristic dyspnoea and cough wakening the patient.

Management

Patients with a productive cough are seldom as disturbed by it as those with a dry irritating cough as in uninfected bronchial tumours, mediastinal obstruction and non-infected chronic bronchitis.

Productive cough

1. The role of the physiotherapist in aiding expectoration and drainage is pre-eminent.
2. Antiobiotics are often useful to clear infection and facilitate easier expectoration. Unscientific as it may appear they are

occasionally useful even when no pathogens have been demonstrated in sputum cultures.

3. Mucolytics, for example bromhexine 8–16 mg tid appear to be useful in spite of the paucity of scientific data to support their use, but only when used regularly for a minimum of four weeks.

Dry cough

A dry cough is undoubtedly helped by:

1. Cough suppressants, e.g.:
    a. Codeine or pholcodeine linctus.
    b. Methadone linctus.
    c. Diamorphine or morphine linctus/solution.
    For cough suppression the dose used is the lowest needed to alleviate this symptom and always so small that depression of respiration is no problem.
2. Humidifying the atmosphere either by steam inhalers or, if oxygen is indicated, by humidification of the gas in the routine way.
3. Steroids (dexamethasone 0.5 mg tid) to reduce oedema surrounding a tumour and relieve bronchial oedema and lessen bronchospasm.
4. Bupivacaine aerosol every four to six hours, provided the patient is capable of steady inhalation of 10 ml of the 0.25% solution on each occasion.

Much confusion appears to exist about the most appropriate nursing techniques. The rules are simple.

1. If the cough is secondary to an uncomplicated bronchogenic carcinoma the patient is seldom comfortable propped bolt upright in bed but better nursed with only two or three pillows. Failure to do this may further embarrass respiration.
2. If due to chronic bronchitis and obstructive airways disease he should be propped up as straight as possible.
3. If there is a pleural effusion (whether necessitating aspiration or not), he should lie on the side of the effusion in a semi-recumbent position. Pleural effusion is often a painful procedure and the doctor must not only be prepared to prescribe appropriate analgesics but remember the problems of nursing a patient on the side of aspiration.

DEPRESSIVE STATES

Many terminally ill patients will be profoundly depressed but not suffering from a 'depressive state' requiring an antidepressant. The injudicious use of an antidepressant may cause unnecessary sedation, worsening of constipation, an unacceptable dry mouth and halitosis and possibly urinary retention on top of all their other problems. *Doctors and nurses must train themselves to differentiate between 'depression' and 'misery' or 'sadness'.* There is substantial evidence that

1. *True depression is under-diagnosed in the terminally ill.*
2. *Most depression is of a reactive type, resulting from inadequately controlled pain and other symptoms.*

The principal features of a depressive state are no different in a terminal illness from those at any other time in life, namely: (a) early morning wakening, (b) disturbed sleep pattern, (c) poor concentration, (d) poor appetite, (e) a sense of guilt or being a burden on others, (f) diurnal pattern. Obviously some of these are also common features of any far-advanced disease, particularly cancer. It may present as agitated anxiety, in the young as well as the old. It is useful to regard the salient diagnostic features as the *changes in sleep pattern* and *impaired concentration* to the exclusion of the others before antidepressants are given a therapeutic trial. Even when features of anxiety are also present it is useful rather to prescribe an antidepressant with anxiolytic properties as the drug of the first choice rather than a simple anxiolytic. Nevertheless, the diagnosis is not an easy one to make and there is often value in giving an antidepressant as a therapeutic trial if the patient is expected to live long enough to benefit from it.

Although there is little to choose between the antidepressants, certain features are worthy of note.

Amitriptyline	Antidepressant/anxiolytic and a useful sedative when taken at night only.
Imipramine	Primarily antidepressant and mildly stimulant – therefore never given after 4 p.m.
Protriptyline	Stimulant antidepressant with no anxiolytic properties.
Clomipramine	Antidepressant but useful when obsessional, ruminative neurotic features are also present.
Trimipramine	Antidepressant with sedative properties. Useful in older, depressed patients with chronic insomnia.
Mianserin	A tetracyclic antidepressant may be effective in 10

days or less but only in a dose of 90 mg nightly (building up slowly from 30 mg).

There are no indications for mono-amine oxidase inhibitors (MAOIs).

It cannot be emphasized enough that the principal form of care must be sympathetic support of the patient with an obvious willingness to encourage him to share his every emotion and express every fear. He will usually benefit from a leisurely chat with a professional more ready to sit and listen than write out a prescription.

DIARRHOEA

True diarrhoea occurs in only 4% of terminally ill patients unless they have such conditions as ulcerative colitis, Crohn's disease, an ileo-colic fistula, or an ileostomy. In most cases it is found to be spurious diarrhoea, hence the aphorism that in terminal care *the commonest cause of diarrhoea is constipation!*

Management

1. Loperamide as required (4 mg tds). This drug has the advantages of speedy action, benefit when taken intermittently on a prn basis, and a regularizing effect on bowel action.
2. Diphenoxylate 5 mg tid.
3. Codeine phosphate 60 mg tds. This useful drug should be used cautiously because it tends to cause loculation of the faeces with the production of hard 'golf balls' liable to produce rectal impaction unless looked for.
4. Steathorrea poses its own problems. Not only is it distressing to the patient but worrying to the relatives because of the additional cleaning of toilet pans and commodes and their fear of infection from the abnormal stool. It is easily controlled with tablets or capsules of pancreatic extract, preferably sprinkled on the food but it can often worsen the nausea and anorexia. It has to be remembered that cholestyramine, so useful for pruritus, worsens steathorrea.

DYSPHAGIA

Patients are usually disappointed that they can swallow very little food but frightened beyond words at the possibility of choking to death or inhaling regurgitated food.

Causes

1. Pharyngeal obstruction (Tumour, extrinsic pressure)
2. Oesophageal candidiasis
3. Oesophageal obstruction
    a. Intrinsic from carcinoma, blocked Celestin tube
    b. Extrinsic from enlarged mediastinal glands
4. Specific neurological disorder (such as motor neurone disease).

Management

1. Treat the primary cause where possible, always being suspicious of candidiasis which may develop very rapidly even in the patient taking nystatin oral suspension by mouth, particularly if he is taking steroids or antibiotics. Ketoconazole may be prescribed along with nystatin if the candida infection is particularly troublesome.
2. Celestin tube for all but totally obstructed carcinoma of oesophagus. Thereafter soft, liquidized foods can be taken easily after a prior drink of soda or tonic water or 1 teaspoon of honey in warm water. The same procedure is repeated after each meal.
3. Dexamethasone 8–12 mg a day for mediastinal obstruction not amenable to radiotherapy or chemotherapy.
4. Skilled nursing to ensure adequate oral hygiene and hydration, correct positioning after meals and reduced air swallowing.

DYSPNOEA

Probably because of co-existent chronic bronchitis in so many men with bronchogenic carcinoma, dyspnoea is severe in 50% of men but is distressing in only 25% of women.

Though less than 1% of patients suffer frightening breathlessness before death it is one of the most feared symptoms because all such patients anticipate death from suffocation and asphyxia. No effort should be spared in attacking this symptom and finding all means to relieve the patient's anxiety which often borders on panic. Having said this, it must be recognized that very little can be done for the underlying pathology in obstructive airways disease, bronchial obstruction by tumour, lymphangitis carcinomatosis and motor neurone disease. On these occasions nothing can replace the reassurance given by a calmly confident nurse or doctor, sitting by the bedside, and both anxiolytics and opiates will always take second place to such sympathy and understanding.

Causes

1. *Caused by cancer*: effusion, atelectasis, consolidation, replacement by cancer of functioning lung, lymphangitis, massive ascites.
2. *Related to treatment*: post-irradiation fibrosis, post-pneumonectomy.
3. *Related to debility*: anaemia, pneumonia, pulmonary embolism.
4. *Un-related to cancer or treatment*: chronic obstructive airways disease, asthma, cardiac failure.

Management

1. *Attempt to modify the pathological process* with antipyretics, corticosteroids, radiation therapy, hormone therapy, chemotherapy, thoracocentesis (if pleural effusion present).
2. Use such *non-drug measures* as a calming presence, cool draught from an open window or fan, breathing exercises, relaxation therapy, hypnosis, and oxygen.
3. *Anxiolytics* such as oral diazepam 2–10 mg each night for sustained effect, or lorazepam 0.5–1 mg sublingually as required. Equally effective as an anxiolytic with the added benefit of calming tachypnoea, use low-dose morphine regularly (morphine solution 2.5–5 mg every 4 hours or MST 10 mg 12-hourly).
4. *Suppress paroxysmal cough* exacerbating dyspnoea with nebulized bupivacaine (10 ml of 0.25% bupivacaine every 4 hours).
5. Panic attacks are best treated with i.v. diazepam (5–20 mg) *or* rectal diazepam solution 20 mg *or* lorazepam 1 mg sublingually.

Oxygen is necessary only for the same indications as at any other time in medical practice, contrary to what some patients and many relatives may feel. The doctor has a responsibility to explain carefully that oxygen will not prolong the life of the patient with lung cancer, nor resuscitate a dying patient.

No medication replaces the reassurance given by the presence of a calm, skilled nurse or doctor.

DYSURIA AND STRANGURY

1. *Urinary tract infection* — already discussed.
2. *Bladder or prostatic carcinoma*, particularly affecting the bladder neck.
3. *Calculi or retained blood clot.*
4. *Infiltration into the bladder of a tumour* from adjacent organs (rectum, cervix, vagina).

In all except urinary tract infection catheterization will probably be necessary in order to perform bladder washouts and deal with incontinence or partial retention often associated with it.

5. *Generalized bladder pain* from a primary carcinoma may be helped by medium dose prostaglandin biosynthetase inhibitors (flurbiprofen 100 mg 8-hourly) but strong analgesics such as the opiates are almost always needed and should not be withheld.
6. *Strangury* is occasionally helped by propantheline 15 mg qid or emepronium 100–200 mg tds. Failure is common and resort may have to be made to permanent catheterization and/or phenol blockade or a coeliac plexus block carried out in hospital/ hospice.

Urinary catheterization

Many ill patients, contrary to expectations, would rather have an in-dwelling catheter than dribbling incontinence or recurring reten-tion. Those who will certainly resent catheterization are patients who at present have no urinary problems but may develop them after certain neurolytic or neurosurgical procedures for intractable pain.

Useful hints for catheter care

1. Use 'Foley' catheters.
2. Do not keep inflating/deflating the bulb or re-inserting different sizes of catheter if the patient develops a urinary leak around the catheter.
3. Only use catheters with bulbs of 5 ml capacity.
4. The simplest bladder washouts are the best in most cases; chlorhexidine 1 in 5000 daily for infection and weekly for maintenance; saline for debris, deposit and clot removal; silver nitrate 1 in 10 000 for distressing bleeding from bladder tumour or mucosa. Daily noxythiolin washouts should only be used

when active antibacterial therapy is called for and bladder lavage with 0.5% acetic or citric acid has failed.

5. The discomfort of catheterization in the anxious patient may be avoided by prior administration of lorazepam 0.5–1 mg sublingually, rectal diazepam solution 10 mg, or dextramoramide 5 mg sublingually (all given 15 minutes prior to the procedure) and liberal use of an anaesthetic gel introduced into the urethra prior to catheterization.

FAECAL INCONTINENCE

This is not only a distressing problem for the patient but a cause for some being admitted to hospital for the sake of relatives.

Cause

1. Lax anal sphincter, particularly in the elderly.
2. Faecal impaction producing spurious diarrhoea.
3. Ano-rectal carcinoma.
4. Excessive intake of laxatives (particulary if containing liquid paraffin).

Management

It is important to do a thorough rectal examination to define the cause. The patient with a lax sphincter may benefit from a constipating agent (e.g. loperamide, codeine phosphate), the constipated patient from appropriate rectal evacuation and regular faecal expanders.

The patient with an ano-rectal carcinoma may be helped by:

1. Radiotherapy;
2. Rectal steroids (e.g. prednisolone suppositories bd, betamethasone foam bd, or a prednisolone retention enema daily);
3. The provision of appropriate incontinence aids;
4. The provision of a portable air freshener.

FUNGATING TUMOURS AND ODOURS

Even when skilled nursing is provided for the patient with a fungating tumour, he will be distressed by any odour because of his embarrassment and its ability to isolate him even further from relatives and friends. Denying the existence of a bad smell will never comfort a patient acutely aware of it! In time, some patients, but not their relatives, may become less aware of the smell.

Management

1. Regular cleaning of the fungating tumour with hydrogen peroxide 3%.
2. Radiotherapy should be considered for all fungating tumours.
3. Antibiotics have a place for reducing secondary infection and discharge. Metronidazole tablets/pessaries/gel are useful when inserted into a sinus or placed on a fungating tumour once daily to remove odour.
4. Charcoal pads are extremely effective on malodorous lesions. They are applied on top of all other dressings in use.
5. Yogurt (plain) applied to deep ulcers/sores helps to de-slough and is reapplied daily.
6. Bismuth and iodoform paste, applied on gauze to a fungating, malodorous tumour, helps haemostasis and reduces odour. It is changed every two or three days.
7. Commercial deodorizers are available and are preferable to hand-held aerosol air fresheners whose scent comes to be associated with painful memories for relatives after the death.

HALITOSIS

This is seldom reported, but often suffered. Patients are often not aware of it and it goes without saying that it is a source of great distress and embarrassment to relatives.

Causes

1. Bad oral hygiene (thrush, dental sepsis, dentures, loss of saliva, mouth breathing, dehydration).
2. Cesspool halitosis because of delayed gastric emptying or a gastric carcinoma (particularly linitis plastica).
3. Carcinomas of mouth, throat, pharynx and bronchus.
4. Sinus and nasopharyngeal infections (usually pre-existent to the terminal disease).
5. Pre-existent bronchiectasis.

Management

1. Energetic attention to oral hygiene in all patients. Dentures MUST be removed and cleaned regularly, preferably in 0.2% chlorhexidine or half-strength domestic bleach.
2. Use of two-hourly lemon and glycerine mouth swabs.
3. Metroclopramide 10 mg qid, or domperidone 10–20 mg qid, to speed gastric emptying.
4. Peppermint or 'Amplex' sweets and lozenges.
5. The odour from a bronchogenic carcinoma may be reduced by metronidazole 200 mg tid by mouth.

HICCUPS

Causes

1. Irritation of the phrenic nerve by tumour involvement at the hilum of the lung.
2. Direct irritation of the diaphragm (infection, tumour).
3. Uraemia.
4. Dyspepsia (especially with hiatus hernia).
5. Elevation of diaphragm (from enlargement of the liver or ascites).

Management

1. Correct uraemia if possible.
2. Simple re-breathing from a paper bag.
3. Haloperidol 0.5 mg qid orally or 1.5 mg intramuscularly during attacks.
4. Chlorpromazine 25 mg qid or prn during attacks (though its sedative effect may distress the patient).
5. Metoclopramide 10 mg qid or domperidone 10–20 mg qid.
6. Hyoscine 0.4 mg prn (but often contraindicated because of its ability to cause distressing tachycardia).
7. Interruption of phrenic nerve is rarely indicated but possible by:
   a. Phenol infiltration of the nerve in the neck under local anaesthetic
   b. Surgical crushing of nerve.

HYPERCALCAEMIA

Hypercalcaemia is a complication commonly associated with multiple bone metastases and less commonly can be caused by the ectopic production of parathormone by a tumour.

Clinical features:

tiredness	anorexia
nausea	vomiting
constipation	thirst
polyuria	drowsiness
confusion	coma
exacerbation of pain	

Management

1. Adequate fluid intake, 2–3 litres daily.
2. Frusemide (40 mg/day).
3. Dexamethasone (2 mg qid).
4. Oral phosphate (when normocalcaemia achieved).
5. Intravenous fluids, phosphate and mithramycin may also be necessary in some patients.

Hypercalcaemia should not be considered in isolation, and how active the treatment should be in an individual patient will depend on how distressing the symptoms are to the patient and whether any further treatment of the malignancy is available and likely to be of benefit.

HYPERHIDROSIS (EXCESSIVE SWEATING)

Patients are distressed by this because of the inevitable discomfort and embarrassment and, though they seldom proffer this reason, by the one-time association with tuberculosis and 'fever'. They occasionally admit they are frightened in case they have another disease infectious to their relatives, in addition to cancer.

Causes

1. Toxaemia associated most commonly with liver metastases.
2. Intercurrent infection. (Except in the *final* days of a terminal illness it is usually worthwhile dealing with an intercurrent infection if by doing so the patient's comfort is ensured.)

Management

1. Try to deal with the cause.
2. Cimetidine 200–400 mg each night, or ranitidine 150 mg each night can be of help.
3. Indomethacin 25 mg qid after meals orally, or 100 mg suppositories bd.
4. Propranolol 40 mg tid. (If not contraindicated because of bronchospasm and cardiac failure.)
5. Steroids (dexamethasone 2–4 mg/day).
6. Most patients are more assisted by skilled nursing, frequent sponging and appropriate advice about clothing and bedding than by any medical measures.

INSOMNIA

This is more commonly reported in advanced carcinoma than in other conditions, is a genuine cause of distress to many patients and their relatives and can eventually become a reason for hospital admission if relatives lose their own sleep.

Causes

The aetiology is ill understood but is usually found to be associated with one or more of the following and each merits attention:

1. *Poorly relieved physical distress* which may not be reported as such by the patient.
2. *Anxiety*, often so mild that it is not apparent during the day.
3. *Depression*. Disturbed sleep pattern may remain the only feature for a long time and failure to explore this and consider a therapeutic trial of an antidepressant is a common mistake.
4. *Nocturia* which may respond to emepronium 200 mg each night.
5. *Night sweats*, particularly in patients with hepatic involvement by tumour, frequently respond to cimetidine 200–400 mg each night or ranitidine 150 mg each night.
6. Previous dependence on barbiturates, benzodiazepines or alcohol which have recently been discontinued for some reason.

Management

All that can be done here is list important points on the commonest used drugs, none of which is ever a substitute for companionship and a carefully tailored atmosphere of safety.

1. When all have been explored one may still be left with no obvious cause. In this case it is wisest to assume that anxiety and/or depression are responsible and every effort be made to explore this and prescribe a sedative antidepressant with anxiolytic properties (e.g. amitriptyline 50 mg or doxepin 50 mg).
2. If barbiturates have been used in the past they should be resumed.
3. The agitated and depressed patient will respond better to pericyazine (10–20 mg) nightly than benzodiazepines or chlorpromazine.
4. The ruminative patient may do better with clomipramine (25–50 mg) nightly.
5. Long-acting benzodiazepines, whilst often aiding sleep, usually leave the patient with daytime sedation and poor concentration which he may find unacceptable. They are nevertheless very useful in terminal care.
6. An alcoholic drink at night, particularly in the elderly and those not accustomed to much daytime alcohol, usually helps.
7. A low wattage lamp left on in the room helps to dispel some of the primitive fears of the dark.

There will remain patients, particularly the older ones in hospital, who have a reversed sleep pattern, awake at night and asleep by day. They must be left with this pattern and the routine of nursing attention adjusted accordingly, every effort being made to reassure the patient and his family that his behaviour is not, as may be imagined, a manifestation of a neurotic or psychotic state, nor a difficult personality manifesting itself.

INTESTINAL OBSTRUCTION

The management of this relatively common condition is a difficult problem for the doctor caring for a terminally ill patient.

General Principles

1. Any treatable cause such as postoperative adhesions and faecal impaction should be excluded.
2. Surgery is indicated when the patient's prognosis is still good and a localized blockage is considered likely.
3. Intravenous fluids and naso-gastric aspiration ('drip and suction') are only appropriate in preparation for surgery, but *rarely* if ever in terminal care.

4. Medical management of the individual symptoms is usually the most appropriate option in the terminally ill patient.

The symptoms and treatment options can be summarized:

1. Colic — loperamide 4 mg prn
regular morphine orally, by suppository, or diamorphine by subcutaneous injection or syringe-driver
coeliac plexus block

2. Visceral pain — morphine orally, by suppository, or diamorphine by subcutaneous injection or syringe-driver
coeliac plexus block

3. Constipation — a faecal softener (docusate, lactulose)

4. Diarrhoea — loperamide 4 mg prn
steroids (dexamethasone 4 mg bd)

5. Vomiting — haloperidol (0.5–1 mg tid orally or by syringe-driver)
cyclizine 50 mg tid
chlorpromazine 10–25 mg tid
steroids (dexamethasone 4 mg bd)

6. Dry mouth — scrupulous oral hygiene, ice to suck, frequent sips of iced fluids

7. Diet — The patient should be encouraged to take a little of what he fancies.

NOTE:

The patient who is dehydrated complains more of a dry mouth than thirst and will be made more comfortable by scrupulous attention to this than by the correction of dehydration and electrolyte imbalance by intravenous fluids.

NAUSEA AND VOMITING

Upsetting as it is, vomiting is less distressing to many patients than persistent nausea and sometimes easier to control. Neither symptom is an inevitable feature of terminal illness. Though nausea may not always be accompanied by vomiting the two symptoms are best considered together.

Causes (not in order of frequency)

1. Drug-induced (narcotics, non-steroidal anti-inflammatory drugs, antibiotics, cytotoxic drugs, digoxin, oestrogens and syrup-based medicines).
2. Constipation.

3. Sub-acute intestinal obstruction.
4. Raised intracranial pressure.
5. Hypercalcaemia, uraemia, septicaemia.
6. Anxiety state (possibly made worse by poorly controlled pain and other symptoms).
7. Cough-induced.

Management

1. Remove or correct the cause where possible. For example, one can change from morphine to methadone hopefully to lessen constipation, change antibiotics, use alternative routes of drug administration, encourage more regular bowel evacuation, manipulate diet, the temperature of food and timing of meals. *It cannot be emphasized enough that opiates seldom cause persisting nausea after four or five days of regular use.*
2. Reduce raised intracranial pressure with dexamethasone (initially i.m. 4 mg qid maintained at 4 mg twice daily orally).
3. Correct hypercalcaemia by maximum fluid intake, dexamethasone 4 mg qid i.m. then orally and thereafter maintain normal plasma levels with a maintenance dose of dexamethasone.
4. Control dysphagia and oesophageal regurgitation with:
    a. antacids — magnesium hydroxide (laxative);
    b. aluminium hydroxide (constipating);
    c. magnesium trisilicate (mildly laxative);
    d. cimetidine or ranitidine by tablet or injection in the same dose;
    e. carbenoxolone (in appropriate form) for oesophageal, gastric and duodenal irritation with due attention to electrolyte balance.
5. Nystatin and/or ketoconazole and/or amphotericin B lozenges for oesophageal candidiasis.
6. ANTI-EMETICS (depending on desired site of action).

CENTRAL ACTION	*GI TRACT*
prochlorperazine	metoclopramide
chlorpromazine	domperidone
promethazine	cimetidine
haloperidol	ranitidine
trifluoperazine	
droperidol	
cyclizine	
hyoscine	
thiethylperazine	

It should be remembered that terminally ill patients seldom like the sedative effects of the central acting anti-emetics, that in a few patients two anti-emetics will be required (one central acting, one gut acting).

7. Should the above measures fail, and nausea persists, it can be assumed that there is a high level of anxiety and/or depression, worthy of a short trial of an intermediate-acting benzodiazepine, e.g. lorazepam 0.5–1 mg tid.

8. In some patients, when all else has failed, no hypercalcaemia or raised intracranial pressure been found, and there are no strong contraindications to its use, dexamethasone will help to control nausea. It is given in a dose of 16 mg on the first day, reducing by 4 mg daily to a maintenance dose of 4 mg per day.

9. Cough-induced vomiting — control cough.

No medical measure will be effective unless adequate emotional support is given to both patient and relatives, because nausea which prohibits eating upsets the family more than anything apart from pain. It is frequently justifiable to admit a patient to hospital to break the circle of nausea and vomiting. Frequently the change of surroundings and a sense of security and empathy will be all that are required.

OEDEMA

Unilateral upper limb

Lymphoedema: A Flowtron or Jobst intermittent compression pump should be tried, starting thrice daily then increasing up to 4-hourly if tolerated by the patient. During the day the patient should wear a firm elastic armlet, preferably tailor made (e.g. Jobst armlet). Elevation of the arm on pillows or in a sling suspended from a drip stand or head of the bed may be effective but is usually uncomfortable because shoulder movements are very limited.

Bilateral upper limb

Superior vena cava obstruction, with venous distension in the area drained by the SVC, infra-orbital oedema and upper limb cyanosis. The management of this with prompt radiotherapy, chemotherapy, or high-dose dexamethasone is dealt with elsewhere.

Unilateral lower limb

The three principal causes in terminal care are:

1. *Venous and lymphatic obstruction* caused by a pelvic tumour. Radiotherapy and chemotherapy should be considered.

2. *Deep venous thrombosis*: The decision whether or not to give anticoagulants is a difficult one requiring a careful assessment of the whole clinical pattern. It is helpful to invite a specialist colleague to share in this decision.

3. *Infection*, whether cellulitis, lymphangitis or deep tissue infection from nearby tumour, treated usually with appropriate antibiotics, bedrest and analgesics as required.

Bilateral lower limb

The three principal causes in terminal care are:

1. *Lymphatic and venous obstruction* by a pelvic tumour, managed by radiotherapy, high-dose dexamethasone (with less success than in SVC obstruction) and diuretics, preferably spironolactone 200–400 mg a day.

2. *Cardiac failure*, treated in the routine way.

3. *Hypoalbuminaemia*, either from dietary deficiency or loss in ascitic fluids. Rarely is it appropriate or possible to correct this in a terminally ill patient.

Frequently lower limb oedema troubles the patient by appearance more than discomfort and is the result of sitting for prolonged periods with the feet dependent. This is not an indication for diuretics, with the resultant need for careful watch on electrolytes, but for elevation of the feet, support stockings, and reassurance that this is not cardiac or renal failure.

PLEURAL EFFUSION

Though not strictly a symptom this complication is common enough to pose a problem to the clinician. The rule is that it should be aspirated only: (a) for diagnostic purposes; (b) if, by so doing, incapacitating dyspnoea will be relieved.

Where the effusion is likely to recur and the life expectancy of the patient is still likely to be long, it is worth considering the instillation into the pleural space of an agent producing pleurodesis.

It is worth remembering that pleural effusion secondary to a bronchogenic carcinoma carries a poor prognosis. On the other hand, patients with breast carcinoma complicated by pleural effusion may still survive many months.

PRURITUS

Causes

1. Pre-existing skin disease (eczema, psoriasis, infestation).
2. Dry skin (particularly senile pruritus).
3. Obstructive jaundice.
4. Melanomatosis.
5. Hodgkin's disease.
6. Anxiety state.
7. Allergic reaction.

Management

In obstructive jaundice it is worth trying:

1. Haloperidol 0.5 mg tid or 2 mg at night.
2. Steroids (dexamethasone 2 mg bd reducing to 2 mg/day).
3. Testosterone 10 mg sub-lingually tid.
4. Cholestyramine 1 sachet bd if the patient can tolerate the taste.

General non-specific measures

These are in addition to treating any pre-existing skin condition.
1. Emulsifying ointments.
2. Sodium bicarbonate washes as often as desired by the patient (one tablespoon of powder in the smallest volume of water sufficient to dissolve it). Patients often report this as more effective than any other measure.
3. Terfenadine 60 mg bd.
4. Chlorpheniramine maleate 4 mg tid or trimeprazine tartrate 10 mg tid but sedation may be unacceptable.
5. One per cent phenol calamine lotion prn.
6. Crotamiton 10% cream prn.
7. Weak topical steroids (1% hydrocortisone).
8. Cold fans playing on the exposed skin or 'eau de cologne' sprays.
Once again, pruritus is more usually helped by skilled nursing than any medical measures.

RECTAL IRRITATION AND DISCHARGE

Both symptoms upset patients by the discomfort they produce. Discharge produces the additional embarrassment of odour, incontinence and extra work for nurses and attending relatives.

Causes

1. Rectal/anal canal carcinoma.
2. Pelvic tumour infiltrating rectal mucosa.
3. Faecal impaction producing faecal leak.
4. Paraplegia with faecal incontinence.
5. Candida infection.

Management

1. Rectal carcinoma should always be considered for palliative radiotherapy.
2. Constant energetic attention to bowel action. In paraplegia and motor neurone disease, it is often useful to constipate the patient and empty the bowel manually twice or thrice weekly. This is sometimes less embarrassing for the patient than a constant faecal incontinence.
3. Lignocaine suppositories bd (remembering that sensitivity to this may develop).
4. Prednisolone suppositories or prednisolone retention enemata bd.
5. When perianal and perineal pain is a problem, but bowel and bladder sphincters are intact, steroids by caudal infiltration reduce symptoms for 8 to 10 weeks. When pain is a problem in a catheterized patient with a colostomy the symptoms can be eradicated by caudal infiltration with phenol 5% in glycerine.

SORE MOUTH

Anything which makes eating or swallowing difficult is worth treating as much for the sake of caring relatives, who feel that feeding the patient is all that is left to them, as for the patient.

Causes

1. Oral candidiasis, present in 75% of patients but often missed

because it presents more commonly as a spongy red mucosa (with angular cheilosis in denture wearers) than the classical white plaques.
2. Aphthous ulcers, much less common.
3. Cytotoxic chemotherapy, in some cases a marked stomatitis may occur.

Management

1. For candidiasis, nystatin oral suspension 1 ml qid is effective only if taken with dentures out at the time, dentures soaked each night in 0.2% chlorhexidine or half-strength domestic bleach, and *maintained until the end of life.*
2. Aphthous ulcers respond to hydrocortisone pellets 2.5 mg qid or carbenoxolone pellets 5 mg or gel qid.
   Both aphthous ulcers and post-chemotherapy stomatitis may be helped with Aschurt's solution (a betamethasone solution) used 4-hourly. This must be prepared freshly for each patient by the pharmacist.
3. Occasionally, even in the absence of proven infection, post-chemotherapy stomatitis improves with cotrimoxazole suspension in the usual dose regime. Given time, it will clear spontaneously.
4. Foods are usually preferred either icy cold or very hot; semi-solids preferred to either fluids or solids.
5. Rarely one resorts to 1% aqueous gentian violet applied hourly with *good* results but ruined linen!

STEROIDS IN TERMINAL CARE

Steroids have many uses in the management of the terminally ill and can prove very beneficial. However, caution must still be used and the dose reduced to the lowest effective maintenance dose as quickly as possible and the drug withdrawn if no benefit is obtained within one or two weeks. They are, in effect, a 'life support' system and their benefits must constantly be weighed against their side effects. (For example, many women in particular will resent the Cushingoid features produced.)

Indications and Doses:

1. raised intra-cranial pressure
   spinal cord compression
   superior vena cava obstruction
   nerve compression
   nerve root compression
   } dexamethasone 4 mg qid initially, reduced as soon as possible to, for example, 2 mg bd.

2. appetite stimulation
   nausea associated with liver
   metastases
   } dexamethasone 2 mg bd initially, reduced to 2 mg each morning.

SUPERIOR VENA CAVA OBSTRUCTION

Though not a symptom nor a common problem, superior vena cava obstruction merits attention because of the extreme distress it can produce and its response to therapy. Every patient with a bronchogenic carcinoma or known mediastinal spread from any tumour should regularly be examined for the earliest signs of its development. Occasionally it may present as one of the emergencies of terminal care.

Management

1. Prompt radiotherapy
2. Cytotoxic chemotherapy
3. Dexamethasone:
   a. Emergency: i.m. 8 mg tid for 2 days reducing to tablets of 20/16/12 mg per day
   b. Maintenance: 8–12 mg per day in divided doses.

URINARY SYMPTOMS

Urinary symptoms are so inter-related that it is appropriate to consider here incontinence, retention, frequency, strangury and cathether problems. Causes and management will be considered together.

Incontinence

1. *Urinary tract infection.* This is worth treating with an appropriate antibiotic if it can be taken orally but intravenous antibiotics are rarely justified in a terminally ill patient. No antibiotic is

justified if the patient has an in-dwelling cathether. It has to be remembered that there may be incidental bacteriuria in old people.

2. *Structural changes in the bladder*, due to tumour and post-irradiation *fibrosis* for which even catheterization may not be wholly successful.

3. *Retention with overflow*, due to spinal cord compression. After the patient has been catheterized the place of laminectomy and/or irradiation should be considered.

4. *Excessive sedation* with hypnotics, tranquillizers, opiates etc.

The occasional patient is helped by emepronium 100–200 mg tds or, if incontinent only at night, by 200 mg on settling.

Urinary retention

1. *Drug-induced*, particularly by anticolinergic drugs, tricyclic anti-depressants, opiates.

2. *Neurological causes*, particularly spinal cord compression.

3. *Faecal impaction* of the rectum.

4. *Prostatic carcinoma* obstructing bladder neck.

Probably all will require a catheter initially, whatever the cause. In '1' it may be possible to withdraw the drug and in '3' evacuate the rectum in the usual way.

WEAKNESS AND LETHARGY

It is axiomatic in good terminal care that each distress is investigated even when, as in this case, the cause is almost certainly the advanced nature of the illness itself. Occasionally one comes across a cause which requires minimal non-invasive investigation and an easy remedy, making all the difference to the quality of the patient's life.

It is therefore useful to investigate:

1. *unnecessary boredom* which can be relieved by skilled occupational therapy, adjustment of relatives' visits, change in environment, and modest useful activities;

2. *excessive sedation or analgesia*;

3. *a true depressive state* which might benefit from an anti-depressant;

4. *hypercalcaemia*, present in 12–15% with advanced cancer (see separate section);

5. *hypokalaemia* with the usual aetiology and again sometimes worthy of correction;
6. *adrenal failure* either because of hypophysectomy, adrenalectomy, tumour deposits in the pituitary adrenals, or failure to take replacement therapy.

3

Emergencies in terminal care

No matter how skilled is the team's anticipation of problems one still encounters genuine emergencies when caring for the dying. Like all emergencies they may occur at any time, require immediate professional attention and demand both therapeutic skills and a sensitive appreciation of the total clinical needs of the patient and family. The unprepared or inexperienced doctor may easily find himself reacting as he might in 'acute' medicine, admitting as an emergency to the receiving hospital, or referring for blood transfusion or other resuscitative procedures, without due regard to the overall condition of the patient, and the needs and the capabilities of the relatives.

SUPERIOR VENA CAVA OBSTRUCTION

This may occur with any condition producing mediastinal adenopathy and in particular the reticuloses, bronchogenic and breast carcinoma. Seldom is it an acute emergency because its development can be followed over days or weeks and may thus be anticipated. Occasionally, however, it develops rapidly and produces intensive dyspnoea, even at rest, and severe enough at night when the patient slips down in bed to suggest paroxysmal nocturnal dyspnoea. Collateral veins become prominent on the anterior chest will, JVP is raised and infra-orbital bags of soft oedema dramatically alter the patient's appearance. The dyspnoea may be alarming and constitute an emergency.

Management

1. When possible the patient should be referred for urgent radiotherapy to the mediastinum. In most areas, general practitioners have direct access to radiation oncologists who will wel-

come a telephone call about such a patient, possibly already well known to them.

2. High-dose dexamethasone, the initial doses given by i.m. injection with a good chance of improvement within 24 to 36 hours, after which it is given orally in reducing doses. The starting dose is 24 mg/24 hours (usually given as 8 mg (2 ml) every hours), reduced by 4 mg per day until the maintenance dose of 2–4 mg per day is achieved.

When radiotherapy is not available, such a regime may achieve almost as good results.

SPINAL CORD COMPRESSION

Not matter how carefully patients with known vertebral metastases are followed up and examined this catastrophe may strike without notice, without trauma. Doctors must be particularly watchful of patients with a malignant deposit, with or without a kyphos in the mid or lower dorsal spine and upper lumbar spine.

The emergency may present as agonizing bilateral nerve root pain radiating from the affected area but more usually is silent. An acute urinary retention develops, varying degrees of weakness, paraesthesia or anaesthesia develop in the legs, and walking becomes impossible. Examination confirms the distended bladder (painful if it is not dystonic), diminution of leg reflexes, power and/or sensation. Frequently there is hyperaesthesia immediately below the affected dermatome and partial anaesthesia over the lumbo-sacral rhomboid.

Management:

1. This is a genuine emergency. If discovered *within* 18 to 24 hours of it happening, neurosurgical decompression may be possible but many neurosurgeons are reluctant to offer it to a patient with a bronchogenic carcinoma because of its poor prognosis. Immediate telephone discussion with a neurosurgical unit is mandatory within this period.

2. Outside this period, or at the suggestion of the neurosurgeon, urgent radiotherapy may achieve good results and immediate referral is called for.

3. When both options are impossible steroids, in the same dose regime as for SVC obstruction, may be very helpful.

4. The acute retention will require immediate catheterization.

VERTEBRAL COLLAPSE

This is similar to spinal cord compression except that severe pain is the principal feature, often unassociated with trauma, made worse by coughing, sneezing and straining. Initially there may be no neurological deficits or sphincter involvement. The housecall will be for intense pain, unlike any experienced in the past by the patient.

Management

1. Admission to the ward/unit where the patient has been investigated is urgently needed, the patient being transported flat, well secured to the stretcher, and covered with an adequate analgesic for the journey.

2. Hospital management will include straight X-rays, possibly myelograms, adequate regular analgesics, and possibly radiotherapy and orthopaedic fixation, all of which should be explained to the patient if possible and certainly the relatives before the patient is transferred.

CONVULSIONS:

These may either be the presenting symptom before the definitive diagnosis is made or the sequel to cerebral metastases from an already diagnosed tumour, usually bronchial or breast. Understandably they are alarming to relatives. In the undiagnosed patient emergency admission is mandatory to define the cause, but in certain circumstances when they occur in a patient already known to have disseminated carcinoma they may be managed at home without resort to hospitalization. Delicate as it may be to do, there is much to be said for forewarning relatives when a patient has been found to have cerebral metastases, particularly if it is felt that they are intelligent and willing enough to help.

Management:

1. When a doctor can be on the scene within minutes, intravenous diazepam (Diazemuls) 10 mg should be administered.

2. When such prompt professional attention is impracticable, relatives can be left with a supply of rectal diazepam solution (Stesolid) and instructed on giving 20 mg at the commencement of

the attack. This will be effective within 15 minutes and last for up to three hours.

Naturally the relatives should be given routine instructions on maintaining an airway, removal of dentures etc. Where prophylaxis is practicable, phenytoin will usually be found the best drug until swallowing becomes difficult when arrangements will need to be made for the community nurse to give daily intramuscular phenobarbitone 100 mg.

HAEMORRHAGE

Fortunately, though haemorrhage is often expected and associated with fatal malignant disease by the lay public, it is seldom severe enough to be classed as an emergency in practice.

Gastric haemorrhage is the most common, often due to gastric carcinoma or following the use of NSAIDs for bone secondaries, or steroids for so many of the other complications of advanced cancer. Some would routinely prescribe an H-2 antagonist but their use as prophylactics is not as yet proven.

Massive haemoptysis is seen less often than might be expected considering the incidence of bronchial carcinoma, probably because of the beneficial effect of radiotherapy in the earlier days of treatment.

Haematuria is very common but usually so persistent in those who have renal and particularly bladder carcinoma and in-dwelling catheters that it seldom upsets patients sufficiently for an emergency call unless with clot retention.

Management

1. The first priority is to sedate the patient who is understandably frightened, his agitation and apprehension striking terror into the helpless relatives. The best drug is diamorphine in a subcutaneous dose of 20–30 mg though *much* larger doses may be required in those already on regular high-dose opiates for pain control. Alternatively the doctor might prefer to give intravenous diazepam 5–10 mg (Diazemuls) by slow injection.

If the patient suffers repeated frightening haemorrhages and the doctor cannot easily get to the patient within minutes he would consider instructing the relatives on the use of rectal diazepam solution (Stesolid) in a dose of 20 mg, leaving the tubes in the house in readiness.

2. The second consideration is whether or not the patient should be admitted to hospital or hospice, not only to reassure him and the relatives, but for possible blood transfusion. Whilst undoubtedly he may feel safer surrounded be professional doctors and nurses and all the accoutrements of a modern hospital, the ambulance journey can be upsetting, there is always the possibility of death within hours of admission with the resultant sense of guilt felt by relatives who wondered if the journey was the cause, and the possibility that he will find himself in a hospital or ward he has never known or come to trust.

More important is the question whether transfusion or 'resuscitation' is appropriate. When there are good reasons for thinking he still has months of good life ahead, such measures may well be justified. When he is already near the end of life and everything until then has been done to enable him to remain at home, such resuscitative procedures are quite unjustified and the doctor must exercise all his clinical skills in making the decision and his gifts of communication and empathy is explaining this decision to the fearful family. Obvious as it may be, it is worth remembering that when he is admitted to hospital he will initially be seen and treated by young, relatively inexperienced colleagues whose training and instinct tell them that all bleeding patients should have an intravenous drip set up and blood given. They should not be put into the position of making such an important ethical decision about a dying patient when the family doctor is more experienced and better qualified to decide.

3. When the haemorrhage is stopped there is usually little point commencing iron therapy unless the patient's general condition suggests he has sufficient time left for him to benefit from it. The discomfort of iron-induced constipation usually outweighs any possible benefits.

HYPERCALCAEMIA

Occasionally this may develop so suddenly as to constitute an emergency. It will show as an acute confusion, weakness, polydypsia and polyuria in a patient apparently reasonably well only days before. In those too confused to ask for drinks or not attended by relatives who appreciate his thirst, he may rapidly become dehydrated and uraemic.

Management

1. The first essential is to rehydrate the patient. He should be enabled to take in at least four to five litres of fluid/day. If this seems impracticable at home and his prognosis appears to be months it will often be easier to refer to hospital for intravenous fluid replacement when the opportunity will probably be taken to add mithramycin.

2. Whether admitted to hospital or not, it will assist to give high-dose steroids and a dose of 24 mg dexamethasone by injection reduced by 4 mg per day to a maintenance oral dose of 2 mg per day, preferably taken in the morning.

3. When the serum calcium (estimated on a specimen taken on the first visit) exceeds 3.5, there is little likelihood that any measures will help the patient. Below that somewhat arbitrary figure, it will be found possible either to maintain him on steroids when he becomes normocalcaemic or transfer him to phosphate (Phosphate Sandos) if he can tolerate this unpalatable preparation.

ACUTE RETENTION

In addition to the usual cause of benign prostatic hypertrophy, retention in the terminally ill may follow opiate administration, the use of tricyclic antidepressants, faecal impaction of the rectum, clot retention in the catheterized patient, and acute urinary infection. Though less common it may be a presenting feature of spinal cord compression.

The management consists of immediate catheterization done by the family doctor (who must therefore always have a small supply of catheters with him). There is no justification for the upheaval of hospital admission merely for catheterization. Subsequently the doctor will try to define the cause and treat accordingly although he will hopefully be reluctant to change from the opiates if they are incriminated.

ACUTE PANIC ATTACKS

The causes are legion and often as difficult for the patient to explain as for the doctor to diagnose. They range from paroxysmal nocturnal dyspnoea and the pain of nerve root compression to the fears created by new lumps, sudden weakness, the terrors of the night or sudden realization of approaching death. They attack those with a reputation for stoicism and calmness as well as those known to the doctors as 'neurotic' or 'emotionally inadequate'. Dying can be a frightening, lonely experience and few of us will blame a patient for reacting in this most understandable way.

Management

1. Before reaching for a prescription pad and ordering a transquillizer, the doctor will take the time needed to find the cause if at all possible. It cannot strongly enough be stated that fears are usually founded on ignorance of what is happening and what *may* lie ahead.

The speck of blood in sputum may be seen as the warning of a massive fatal haemorrhage; sudden dyspnoea may be seen as death from asphyxia, dysphagia as choking, forgetfulness or muddleness as incipient mental illness, pain as the beginning of an agony even the trusted family doctor will be unable to control and so forth.

There is no substitute for the reassurance that comes from the bedside presence of a family doctor or nurse who shows that he or she cares by the way he sits and listens with patience and studied calm.

2. The best drug for a severe attack is intravenous diazepam, 5–10 mg, or intravenous lorazepam 1–2 mg, particularly useful because of its amnesic effect.

3. It is often found helpful to leave some patients with a small supply of lorazepam to be sucked sublingually in a dose of 0.5–1 mg at the commencement of recurrent panic attacks.

4. If the attacks become more frequent and all obvious causes are being competently dealt with, there is then a case for continuous tranquillizing. In this case the doctor will wish to consider low-dose opiates (unless the patient is already on them for analgesia), remembering their adverse effects of constipation, inactivity drowsiness and, after months of use, their dysphoric effect. Alternatively he will look at the longer benzodiazepines and consider diazepam 10 mg nightly, probably a preferable drug in such cases to methotrimeprazine (Veractil) with its undesirable sedation but undoubted analgesic benefit.

5. Such attacks are usually less frequent when the patient has close at hand someone, whether a relative, friend or a professional attendant, whose calm demeanour reassures and inspires tranquillity and confidence.

4

Diet

It would be easy to dismiss this subject with the comment that by the time a patient enters the final months of life all that matters is that he eats a little of what he likes and is able to take. This is, generally speaking, correct but it is not what either the patient or his family want or expect to be told.

For years he has been led to believe that dietary habits influence the development and management of certain diseases and that some foods have therapeutic powers. He cannot be unaware of the claims made for some dietary regimes said to be capable, if not of curing cancer, certainly of bringing about worthwhile remissions.

Even when caring relatives do not subscribe to such ideas, they will nevertheless be anxious to provide a diet capable of maintaining, if not extending, life in the loved one. His persisting anorexia may be seen as a mark of their failure to present attractive and appropriate meals, his intractable nausea as proof of their culinary inadequacy. His weight loss is seen as resulting from inadequate intake of 'good' food in spite of all the luxuries they are buying to tempt him. Preparing meals may be all that is left for them to do to demonstrate their love and devotion.

Experience suggests that there are frequently made mistakes in this matter of diet for the terminally ill.

1. *Avoidance of the subject*. The doctor or nurse may choose to ignore the subject, never giving either patient or relative the opportunity to raise the topic. Even worse is the doctor avoiding the subject and leaving the community nurse to face the questions when even she may not feel confident to answer them. The result may be the patient being pressurized into trying to eat food which is too rich, milk-based 'invalid' foods which may increase nausea and almost certainly will exacerbate constipation, or 'quack' diets which have been reported in the popular press.

2. *Suggesting inappropriate dietary regimes*. Here one thinks of those same invalid diets which, though often useful and possibly all

he may be able to digest, are usually singularly unpalatable and boring. There is the notion that an exceedingly high intake of ascorbic acid (10 g daily) has a beneficial effect on malignant disease when, in fact, it does nothing at that dose except produce diarrhoea. (There is, however, the possibility that 1 g per day may temporarily improve appetite as an alternative to steroids.)

3. *Ignoring proven dietary facts.* Common sense dictates that the patient with a Celestin or Atkinson tube for oesophageal carcinoma be told to take a liquidized diet or at least 'everything you can normally eat from a spoon', avoiding white bread, breakfast cereal lacking in roughage, and lumpy portions of anything. These same patients should be advised to have a glass of mineral water beside them, taking a drink before and after each meal and a mouthful between portions. Even better is to preface the meal with a tea-spoon of honey dissolved in warm water to lubricate the tube.

More common is the problem of constipation (see Chapter 2) and the wealth of dietary advice needed both to prevent it and to treat it.

4. *Presuming that dietary regimes are understood by everyone.* Few patients appreciate that milk is, for the terminally ill, more palatable when diluted with equal parts of soda water and drunk cold straight from the refrigerator, or that a dry mouth is helped by sucking ice-cubes even when the patient is scarcely able to swallow.

Uncooked apple may constipate because of its pectin content whereas stewed or baked apple may be laxative because of the added sugar.

Scrambled egg may be acceptable and palatable when eggs in any other form are nauseating or dyspepsia-inducing.

More important however are the principles that 'little and often' and 'what you fancy when you fancy' bring more comfort than anything else. The doctor is duty bound to explain that the patient's body nearly always knows best about food and seems to know little or nothing about fluid requirements. If he fancies porridge at night he should have it, or ice-cream four-hourly or ice-cubes made from his favourite tipple, provided all helpings are small, imaginatively served, at the temperature that his body prefers, offered on the smallest available plate.

5. *Giving of complicated dietary advice.* As with everything else to do with terminal care, it must never be assumed that the advice given is immediately understood nor readily remembered. It is usually better, should it be the case, to state categorically and repeatedly that there are no 'rules' and he may take whatever he

fancies or to write a list of recommended foods and fluids and a short, undaunting list of 'not recommendeds'.

Particularly is this necessary for the patient who has had to be on a strict regime in the past and now gains nothing from abiding by it. Few cardiac patients in the final weeks of life need be kept on a totally salt-free diet, nor hypercalcaemic patients denied milk. The terminally ill cancer patient may be unable to take the high bulk/bran diet he has grown accustomed to for his diverticular disease.

GUIDELINES FOR DIETARY ADVICE

1. 'Little and often of whatever he fancies' must head the list, with the explanation that his likes and dislikes may change dramatically, not only from day to day but from what he has always preferred in the past. The 'sweet tooth' may now reject everything sweet and choose strong-tasting savouries. The elderly patient who has always regarded ice-cream as a treat for children may find it is the only food his nausea will tolerate.

2. The nearer the end of life, the colder will most patients prefer their drinks, finally accepting crushed ice-cubes to suck when drinking from a glass or feeding cup is impossible.

3. Bright-coloured drinks and tastefully garnished foods are often more attractive and enticing than bland ones. Ice-creams may have a teaspoon of liqueur poured over them or fruit sauce. Steamed fish, mashed potatoes or liquidized foods can be garnished with a tiny sprig of parsley, a dash of tomato sauce or a minute portion of spinach.

4. Careful attention to the choice of cups and crockery will further help. The smaller the plate, the less daunting does the helping appear, particularly if it has a rim to lessen spillage. Cups should be light enough for the frail hands to hold, with handles which will hold deformed or weakened fingers. Feeding cups should have twin handles, straws be corrugated to allow bending and spoon handles be padded to facilitate holding.

5. The person needing most advice and understanding is usually not the patient but the caring relative who dreads failing, despairs when all she offers is rejected or returned, and has not the experience or possibly the culinary imagination to ring the changes.

6. The only proven 'tonic' for the anorexic patient and even then effective for a few weeks only, is a steroid. One may either try

prednisolone 5 mg tid or dexamethasone 2 mg each morning. Traditional over-the-counter 'pick me ups' are useless and their failure will only serve to depress further both the patient and his family.

7. The family doctor, as with everything else he does in terminal care, must share his advice with community nursing colleagues and vice-versa.

5

Aids, appliances and equipment

The home care of the terminally ill does not require any specialized equipment which might not also be useful for patients at any other time in the course of a serious illness or with failing functions. Obvious as this may seem it is worth reminding relatives who may be daunted by the 'special' problems they now face.

Many of those listed below are commonly available in local community nursing stores, others may be obtainable from specialist departments and others again are increasingly being purchased by the more progressive large group practices and health centres throughout the country.

SPECIAL MATTRESSES

The prevention of pressure sores is a major nursing problem in the terminally ill. No one piece of equipment has been found which meets the ideal and nothing (and this bears repeating) replaces the skilled and regular attention of a community nurse or relatives taught the technique of skin care.

As adjuvants to this nursing care, the professionals involved may decide to provide a ripple or bubble mattress, the former having transverse ridges which inflate and deflate in turn to prevent the patient's weight being directed for long on any one area. The latter, the bubble mattress, is possibly superior with its surface of palm-sized bubbles of air. More expensive but thought by most terminal care specialist nurses as the best appliance is the range of Spenco mattresses and chair cushions, easy to wash and exceedingly comfortable for patients.

An alternative for chairs and wheelchairs is the Ro-Ho cushion, ugly and uncomfortable in appearance, but very acceptable to many patients when it is correctly inflated for the individual patient.

SHEEPSKIN COVERS

Usually made not of sheepskin but of synthetic fibres, these come in sizes to cover the whole bed or the area of pressure where the patient lies. They are easily washed but many patients, particularly those perspiring with toxic illnesses, find them too hot. Obvious as it may sound they must be directly under the patient and not covered with sheets or cushions.

TRIANGULAR (DELTA) PILLOWS

These firmly filled pillows are a boon to the dyspnoeic patient who otherwise slips down off his stacked pillows or cannot afford the number of pillows his condition merits.

TABLE FAN

The effect of a fan gently blowing cold air around the dyspnoeic patient can only be psychological but is none the less real and appreciated. He can control it for himself to obtain fresh air, cool himself or blow away odours. It is particularly valuable for patients with bronchogenic carcinoma or cardiac failure.

DEODORIZERS

Whilst the foul smells of most fungating tumours may be adequately controlled with charcoal pads (Denidor, Actasorb), and the smells of ostomy appliances reduced by employing the special charcoal inserts advised by the manufacturers, there remain the patients who have vaginal or rectal discharges, head and neck tumours, and exceptionally foul smelling bowel motions. Not only is the sickroom nauseating, but the smell may so pervade the house that relatives begin to doubt if home care is really possible.

For such patients, the answer rarely lies with aerosol air fresheners whose odour can itself be nauseating or embarrassing for the patient and whose scent will forever be associated with the suffering and death of the patient in the memory of the relatives.

Better to provide a portable, electric deodorizer or, if it is obtainable, an ultra-violet deodorizer appliance fitted to a wall or cupboard.

TOILET APPLIANCES

Commodes are freely available in most parts of the country but the member of the care team ordering one must first decide on the model required. Should it have a back, arms (fixed or removable), castors? Who will take responsibility for instructing the relatives on its cleaning and disinfecting? Have they been reassured that the urine or faeces do not carry the disease (even cancer)?

The frail patient who is still able to use the household WC may need to have a foam rubber WC seatpad provided or handrails to enable him to rise unaided and for the latter equipment the community occupational therapist may have to be called in (and usually finds several other aids which can make all the difference).

BATH AIDS

In practice many patients are keen to bath without the help of community nurses and, though finding it relatively easy and safe to get into the bath, are at risk when attempting to get out of it. For them a handrail either at the side or affixed to the taps is useful, again provided by the occupational therapy services. Almost all will benefit from a non-stick mat, a hair-rinse shower affixed to the taps and a 'back-scrubber' to help them feel independent.

WHEELCHAIRS

Understandably many patients are reluctant to accept the provision of a wheelchair, regarding it as a sign of invalidism and defeat and often by the time they agree to it, it is almost too late for them to get any benefit. The members of the primary care team are ideally placed to persuade him to use one to permit greater mobility both within the house and outside too, particularly if there is someone to push it. The centre responsible for its provision will usually require a doctor's certificate and the measurements of patient's height, length of thigh and breadth of hips. When the patient is particularly obese, this should be reported and some estimate given of weight.

NYLON LADDER

This simple device with wooden bars linked, like a ladder, by nylon ropes can be tied to the bottom of bed or bedframe to enable the patient to pull himself up in bed without troubling a relative. It serves the same purpose as a 'monkey pole' which may require a special bed or fitting and looks more obtrusive.

INTERMITTENT COMPRESSION SLEEVES

These inflatable sleeves, powered by a pump similar to that used for ripple/bubble mattresses, are available for arms and legs. The commonest make in Britain is the Flotron model. Initially it is applied for twenty minutes daily, then twice-daily, then gradually increased up to 30 minutes three or four times daily to relieve lymphoedema. They are only effective used for several days or weeks and, naturally, only appropriate if it is considered that some lymph channels remain patent or the limb can be moved sufficiently for an inflated sleeve to be worn in comfort. They are usually obtainable from physiotherapy departments.

TALKING AIDS

Though more strictly a 'communication' aid, the simplest and cheapest is the chart on which the aphasic patient can point to his need, signified by drawing, e.g. a urinal, glass of water etc.

The most sophisticated, and of especial value for the patient with the bulbar form of motor neurone disease, is the Possum obtainable on special request via the local rehabilitation and neurology services. It is expensive, requires skilled technical fitting, and must be ordered early enough in the patient's decline to be mastered by him to be of any use.

LIQUIDIZER

Many patients, and not only those with Celestin or Atkinson tubes in place for oesophageal carcinoma, may benefit from taking liquidized food provided it is imaginatively served. If the patient cannot affort to purchase a small simple model it can often be borrowed from community stores.

TV/RADIO

A TV with a remote control can assist many patients without the necessity of calling a relative to change channels.

If the patient can manage earphones or earplugs to listen to radio or cassettes or can be provided with a pillow phone placed on, or under, a pillow he may listen to his favourite music without disturbing others. They are cheap and obtainable from most radio shops.

FIRE-RESISTANT APRONS

The patient who insists on smoking either in bed or in his chair when he can scarcely hold his cigarette or keeps falling asleep can be a danger to himself and a cause of much anxiety to his family. This apron can be spread across the bed or his knees. It is obtainable from Tutor Safety Products, Sturminster Newton, Dorset DT10 1BZ.

SYRINGE-DRIVERS

These have been referred to in Chapter 1 and can occasionally be the means of keeping a patient at home who might otherwise have required admission because of the frequency of injections needed. They are obtainable from Graseby Medical, Graseby Dynamics Ltd, Units 3 and 4, Odhams Trading Estate St Albans Road, Watford Herts WD2 5JX.

NEBULIZERS

Their use with bupivacaine has been described in Chapter 2. Used with water rather than bupivacaine they can assist the patient who

Table 6 Using a TENS (transcutaneous electrical nerve stimulator)

1. Connect electrodes to TENS.
2. Moisten electrode 'paddles' with tap water.
3. Place 1 paddle over spinal processes 2 dermatomes above affected dermatomes and affix firmly using strong non-allergenic surgical adhesive tape.
4. Place the other 'migrating' paddle over the worst area of pain and again affix securely.
5. Switch on TENS, starting at lowest voltage and lowest frequency.
6. Slowly increase voltage until patient describes 'tingling' ('like a little electric shock') feeling. If this does not occur at highest voltage, slowly increase frequency until it occurs.
7. At point of 'tingling' minimally reduce frequency and voltage until sensation stops and wait 5–10 minutes.
8. When sensation recurs, again reduce minimally and leave TENS set at that voltage and frequency.
9. Leave *in situ* for 48 hours.
10. After 48 hours use TENS for 4 hours followed by 4 hours off, 4 hours on etc.
11. As site of pain moves, keep spinal electrode in place (re-moistening frequently) and alter site of wettened migrating electrone.

needs humudification to aid expectoration of tenacious sputum. They are obtainable from R.L. Dolby & Co Ltd, Monitor House, Anderson Street, Dunblane SK15 9AJ.

TRANSCUTANEOUS ELECTRICAL NERVE STIMULATORS (TENS) (Table 6)

Useful for grade 2 and 3 pain, post-herpetic neuralgia and the diffuse, vague aches of 'fibrositis', 'lumbago' and cervical spondylosis, these may be purchased from, amongst many suppliers, Andrew Stephens & Co., 41 Dickson Road, Blackpool, FY1 2AP.

6

Communicating with the patient

It is tempting to assume that by the time a patient is receiving 'terminal care' he has already had the diagnosis explained, has accepted it, and now only needs to be kept up to date with what is happening. If only the problem and the challenge were so simple.

There is a danger that the subject of 'telling' can be over-simplified as if there were a set of rules and procedures which, provided the doctor follows them, will obviate any later difficulties. On the one hand we encounter those who would tell 'the truth, the whole truth and nothing but the truth' immediately the diagnosis was confirmed no matter what the prognosis, treatment options or implications. At the other extreme are the colleagues who work on the thesis that if a patient asks he should be told; if he does not, he should not be told because he clearly does not want to know. The author happens to believe that neither practice is particularly helpful because each is over-simplistic. The area between is grey, dangerous as a minefield but has to be trodden. If there are any useful generalizations they can only be that 'telling' very often turns out to be 'confirming', that denial can be a useful defence mechanism; that almost every patient swings between accepting and denying; and that the doctor is seldom if ever justified in telling a downright lie though he may often have to demonstrate consummate skill and compassion in the way he slowly infuses the truth to his patient.

PROBLEMS OF COMMUNICATING

Obvious as they may be to many experienced doctors and nurses, it might be profitable to look at some of the problems of communicating the diagnosis in the *early* days because many of the problems of communication during the terminal phase are related to them.

The full explanation may not have been understood or remembered

We are all aware (or ought to be) of how little is accurately remembered by a patient after what was intended to be a simple, straight explanation in the surgery or consulting room. Usually no more than two out of five points can be recalled. If the word 'cancer' was in the first sentence, probably nothing else was remembered – no details of the optimistic prognosis, possibilities of treatment and so forth. Other patients have such highly developed denial and defence mechanisms that immediately they erased from memory the sinister part of the explanation and heard and remembered only those sections related to treatment. 'I recall the specialist talking about operations and radium but he didn't ever say it was serious!'

The same applies to any attempt which was made to give a prognosis. The patient tends to go to one extreme or the other. 'He clearly said that in his experience I could have up to two years' though his wife may have equally clear recollection that what was in fact said was '... anything from two months to two years'. At the other extreme is the patient who only remembers the 'two months' and long after these have elapsed because of the success of the initial treatment lives in terror lest each day be his last because he is convinced he is living on borrowed time.

The language used by the doctor may not have been understood

'I was never told I had cancer! You quite clearly said I had a tumour.' How commonly one encounters a patient who temporarily thrives with a partially resected tumour in him because the surgeon said — 'I cut out everything I could see' but did not add that distal metastases were found or deposits found in liver or nodes.

Our attempt to describe sinister pathology in euphemistic terms is commendable but can so easily lead to further misunderstandings when the description was not understood or, as so frequently happens, other medical and nursing colleagues use different terms or analogies. 'He explained I had soft areas in my bones and the next one I saw spoke of little seeds from that cancer I had years ago — now I don't know who to believe!' 'One told me I had swelling of my brain and it would be cured with these tablets but the next said the tablets were only meant to help and not cure.' The possibilities for different explanations and hence everdeepening misunderstanding by the patient are legion.

Well recognized as it should be by most doctors it is worth reminding ourselves that non-medically educated people have very little understanding of their anatomy and physiology. We are foolish to imagine that they either know where the liver is or anything about its function. A description of an 'inflammation of the liver' may be taken as nothing more serious than a mild dyspeptic episode or a potentially fatal attack of hepatitis. 'Bronchitis' may be a description of a minor chest complaint of little import or, if relatives have been known to suffer and die from it, a sentence of death.

The word of the hospital doctor may be regarded as infallible

The apparent optimism of the surgeon who 'took it all away' has been referred to. Is he wrong at that stage to withhold the information that nodal involvement and distal spread were found? Would it help if he burdened the patient in the early postoperative days with the information that most patients succumb to disseminated carcinoma within such and such a period no matter how 'successful' was the operation? That patient, on returning home after surgery, expects his family doctor to share and reiterate the consultant's optimism and enthusiasm and not to describe anything in any way different or more threatening.

The changing prognosis may be withheld from or not understood by the patient

As doctors we do not sufficiently appreciate how the hopes and fears of our patients wax and wane with the relapses and remissions of so many diseases. This pattern is likely to become more and more a feature of our care programmes in the future.

A good example is the patient with breast carcinoma. When the lump is found and its malignant nature explained to her as it must be, she is understandably frightened possibly to the point of despair. Years may elapse before recurrence occurs, during which time she increasingly puts it to the back of her mind though, let us remember, she does *not* forget it. Every single illness or period of malaise or lethargy raises unspoken fears of its return. The shorter the illness the easier it is for her to be confident her fears were unfounded; the longer the illness, the more vague her doctor's explanations or the more detailed and prolonged any investigations, the worse are her forebodings. When it eventually recurs her fears return and may only slowly recede again as the months pass after further surgery and radiotherapy. Each new course of treatment, whether surgery, radiotherapy or chemotherapy, heralds a new evaluation of her prognosis. Each time *she* may wonder if this is the final phase but her medical attendants know otherwise but fail to keep her informed. The paradox here is that such ladies may find it well-nigh impossible to accept when the final phase *does* come and 'terminal care' is instituted, so often has she been there in her own mind only to find that the doctors always had something else they could do. 'Why can't they do any more now?'

A similar picture could be described for patients with chronic respiratory disease frequently complicated by intercurrent infection necessitating ever more sophisticated antibiotic therapy in hospital or for cardiac patients who for years teeter on the brink of death and cannot believe it when finally no more active treatment is available to them.

TELLING THE PATIENT

In a handbook on Domiciliary Terminal Care it is obviously not appropriate to dwell at any greater length on this problem of 'telling' when the diagnosis is made except perhaps to reiterate certain fundamental questions. In the author's opinion the most important is not 'Should a patient be told?' but rather:

Who should tell?

The answer must surely be the doctor who best knows the patient, has the best relationship with him and is in possession of sufficient facts about his condition and the pathogenesis of the disease to do it well. This may be the family doctor or the hospital consultant but, whichever one it is, there must be adequate consultation between them before and after the patient is informed to ensure the best communication between the professionals and the patient, and between all the professionals themselves.

How should the patient be told?

Should it be in a single interview or by slow infusion of the information over days, weeks or months? Should he be told it is serious and the fuller significance be reinforced and explained as the passing of time brings it home to the patient? If euphemisms or analogies are used they should be quoted verbatum in letters between professionals. 'I did not state explicitly he had metastases in the spine but rather that he had many softened areas in his bones due to his cancer/tumour/disease we treated in 1980 . . .'.

Where should the patient be told?

Should it be in a bed in the middle of a busy ward or in a consultant's office or in the GP's surgery? Should it be in the safety of his own home, alone or surrounded by his loved ones?

Should the relatives be told first?

There is no doubt that, strictly, relatives have no *right* to be told something about a patient no matter how much they love him and wish to protect him. Almost without exception they will place an embargo on his being told the truth and it is a brave doctor who will then feel able to go against their wishes, much as he may appreciate the problems which will then lie ahead for everyone, not least the relatives. This is one of those many occasions in medical practice when, ethical principles aside, there can be no hard and fast rules. If the patient is told and then proceeds to deny all knowledge he has been given, what has the doctor to do with and for the relatives on whom much of the burden of caring will fall? If the family is informed and the patient left in ignorance, how is each to be supported through their quite different needs and crises? Can they maintain this conspiracy of silence and for how long? Would it permit the doctor to give the best possible care to the patient if he is fettered with restraints? For the general practitioner it poses a particular problem—that of coping with the grief of relatives who are expecting the death, living daily in the shadow of it and must live a life of deceit with someone they have never knowingly deceived in a long and happy marriage.

It has been suggested that 'do you tell the patient' is not the most important challenge to the doctor. This is certainly the case for old patients who are rarely keen to know the exact diagnosis but rather if, like so many of their family and friends, their time has come. It matters little to them whether the system which is failing is the cardiac or the respiratory. What *does* matter—and they both need to know and have a right to know—is how their comfort may be maintained, whether they may be able to remain at home, who will look after them and whether or not their dignity will be respected as they would wish.

When a young person is found to have a potentially fatal condition there is once again no possible debate about whether or not to inform him. The young woman with leukaemia must be fully and repeatedly informed and kept up-to-date if she is to receive months or years of aggressive chemotherapy. No matter how optimistic the doctor may be about the eventual treatment for a young man with a malignant teratoma, he will have to know what lies ahead. The middle-aged man, so well until a month ago, and now found to have a small cell bronchogenic carcinoma cannot be fobbed off with an explanation about 'influenza' if his prognosis, even with modern chemotherapy, is less than two years much of which will be spent in and out of hospital for his cytotoxics. Even the man with a squamous cell bronchogenic carcinoma who is not a candidate for chemotherapy and may not, at least in the early stages, need palliative radiotherapy, cannot be kept in ignorance of his condition when, all too soon, he finds his health deteriorating and needs to know why, needs to settle his affairs, needs to prepare himself and his family, and needs to feel he can trust his doctor implicitly.

What of the patient who is not told?

One of the most important discoveries of recent years is that almost all patients find out for themselves what is happening. They do this in a variety of ways:

1. They suspect a sinister diagnosis, often before the definitive diagnosis has been made. Particularly is this the case when relatives or friends have had similar symptoms or investigations, when investigations were protracted, or the explanations that were given were vague. So common is it the practice of doctors to be totally frank and explicit when describing a *benign* condition that any vague, nebulous description is seen by patients for what it is – a well-intentioned attempt by the doctor to shield him from something intensely frightening and threatening.

2. They suspect when doctors themselves appear embarrassed, ill at ease or nervous when speaking to them. Do we need to be reminded that all the time we are studying our patients they are also studying *our* expressions, *our* body language, *our* eyes avoiding their gaze?

3. They notice the change in relatives — sadness, strain, embarrassment, discomfiture, secrecy, distancing — and realize that they know something not disclosed to the patient. As the patient in hospital said: 'Why did my wife come in late to visit me, the

first time she had ever been late, and sit rubbing her eyes reddened with conjunctivitis when she had never had it before that day?' The patient upstairs in his bedroom knew something was sadly wrong when his wife talked for so long downstairs with the family doctor then came upstairs red-eyed and strained.

4. The return of distant relatives tells its own tale. How is it possible for the young plumber son to be able to drop in to see his father en route to America from Australia on a business trip when father had to pay his fare out to Australia only six months previously?

5. Patients look inside case notes when the doctor leaves them on the hospital bed or on his surgery table. Others listen more attentively than we realize to the bedside tutorial of medical students or spot the panic which flashed across the face of the young House Doctor or nurse when he spoke of not getting better.

6. Our patients swap stories and experiences every bit as often in medical wards as in surgical or gynaecology wards. They know where the cancer units are, what radiotherapy is for, why people go into hospices or Marie Curie Homes.

In the opinion of the author it is vitally important to recognize not only the problems and pitfalls of imparting the knowledge and details of the diagnosis, but also to remember the strong possibility that, whether explicitly told or not, he will have had his suspicions often from the earliest days. Seldom is ignorance bliss!

THE FINAL PHASE

Let us now progress to the final phase when terminal care is called for and doctor and nurse must work together to ensure not only comfort of body but peace of mind.

What does the patient want to, need to, know?

Probably the commonest question would be how long he has left to him. How frequently it is asked by patient or relative with the same words 'I know it is silly of me to ask, and probably you can't say, but do you know how long?' The inexperienced doctor easily falls into the trap of trying to give a deliberately vague prognosis but even this can be hazardous. If he says 'weeks' it is assumed that he means seven or less because otherwise he would have said 'months'.

If he says 'months' it must be much less than a year or he would have said so or fixed the time by some festival such as Christmas or Easter. Whatever is said is almost certainly going to be taken literally, clung to by the patient or family, or used to influence family members to return from the far corners of the globe. No matter how often the question is asked, very few people use the information to any advantage. No matter how vehemently the doctor explains that he is doing little more than guessing, the layman continues to believe that doctors have some secret scientific means of determining the prognosis, little realizing how we calculate it on the subjective reports from the patient as much as on any objective data we have, until the final week or so. It cannot be over-stressed that the safest statement, for the patient and all the professional attendants, is that couched in the most general terms without any attempt whatsoever at predicting a time. 'Time is certainly short – he is going to get progressively weaker and more weary.'

He will most certainly want to know, even if he does not say so explicitly:

'What will I have to suffer?'

Here the doctors and nurses are on strong ground. They can explain that, whatever pain there *may be*, it can be controlled, the dyspnoea can be reduced, insomnia beaten, appetite helped and loneliness guarded against. It is worth repeating what is said elsewhere in this handbook that patients fear such things as choking, suffocating, insanity, incontinence, loss of dignity and privacy, and increasing dependency. They have every right to expect their attendants to know this and to know whether their illness will produce any of them and then be reassured that the attendants have the necessary experience and skills to fight them.

'Will I have reason to be frightened?'

Is it sufficiently appreciated by doctors and nurses that the greatest dread of each dying patient is fear itself? Many people have never known fear, have no idea whether or not they will be able to cope with it or even express or explain it. Fear is usually fed by the unknown. *Truth and information are the antidotes to fear.* They do not ask for or need all the knowledge of their condition which is possessed by the doctor or nurse. They *do* need to have every question answered honestly, every fear ventilated, every respect shown for their intelligence.

'Are you just trying to keep me alive?'

Obvious as it is to the professionals that all efforts are now aimed at palliation and not either cure or prolongation of life it cannot reasonably be expected that the patient will understand that. In particular, this is the case when the number of his medications increases, more colleagues are called in, admission to hospital is suggested, or temporary improvement begins to look to him like a remission starting. He may regard antibiotics as life-saving drugs and need to have it explained that in him they are only to aid his breathing or reduce the discomfort of cellulitis around the fungating tumour.

The terminally ill patient is rarely if ever upset to have described how all efforts are aimed at his comfort. After what may be months or years of illness he may be profoundly upset if he believes his doctor does not recognize or accept that he is dying and is now trying to prolong a life which has lost much of its quality.

'Will you send me back to hospital?'

Only the much-trusted family doctor can answer this because only he will know the strengths and weaknesses of the family, the patient's attitude to the hospital, what care is needed and whether the hospital is able/willing to have him back for terminal care, whether the family would be able to spend as much time as they would want with him and what *their* feelings would be about his leaving their care.

Once again, as in so many cases in this chapter, would it be dangerous to be dogmatic in advice or in the response to the patient. Even the most skilled and experienced family doctor cannot forecast what will happen from day to day. Today's comfortable patient may tomorrow have a spinal cord compression, intractable pain, or uncontrollable left ventricular failure. The strain on the community nursing service may tell or a partner or locum see the home situation quite differently.

Better to answer this question with a question. 'What do you want yourself?' Experience strongly suggests that more people than we realize would prefer to remain at home but, as the end approaches, they become more and more aware of the additional work and strain for the family and visiting attendants. Occasionally they request, or hope for, admission for their own sakes. More commonly they do so for the sake of others and then is the primary care team challenged to ensure that everything possible is being done for the *family* and every additional resource called in. This may mean Marie Curie night nurses, Macmillan nurses to advise and support, all necessary aids and equipment provided in good time *before* crises develop.

If a patient hopes to return to a familiar hospital where he is well known and whose staff he respects, it should be promised to him and the ward contacted in good time to appraise them of his decline.

If he would prefer to remain at home he can be told how every possible effort will be made to enable him to do so and only if something happens which calls for 'more hands available to help you' will he be sent back.

Two things remain to be said on this subject. The first is that such patients should not, if it can possibly be avoided, be sent into a strange hospital via the Bed Bureau. They have more than enough to worry them and create fear and apprehension without having to relate a history to a new medical and nursing team and then build up a relationship of trust with people they have never known before. The second thing is that admission to hospital is often seen by relatives as a reflection of their failure or inadequacy. At all costs the family doctor must explain that they have done a wonderful job (whether they have or not) and might have been able to carry on doing so but now they need more hands to lift him, people there at night, extra nurses to give injections when they are required, and time in their own beds to keep up their strength for what still lies ahead. In most people's grief there is an element of guilt. The doctor and nurse can do much to reduce this feeling by the sensitive and sympathetic explanation of why the patient may have to leave home.

'How will I die?'

Behind this uncomfortable question, asked quite frequently if the patient is enabled to feel free enough to ask it, are the unspoken questions of whether he will be conscious and aware of what is happening, whether it will come suddenly, whether he will get any warning, whether he will be alone, whether he will fight for breath, bleed or convulse. The doctor and nurse can usually answer with confidence that as the time approaches he will become more tired, sleep much more and never be left alone at any time. They can say with honesty that he will not struggle for breath, nor endure pain. Unfortunately this description of death as like a peaceful sleep may have the opposite effect on some patients who will then fight off all sleep and strive to stay awake in spite of every sedative tried by the doctor!

The reader will not need to be reminded that most terminally ill patients ask few of these questions directly. They may ask them indirectly, casually bring them into conversation, phrase them as though they were actually being asked by others or never mention them at all. Few patients talk much of what lies ahead, fewer still ask many questions and many manage to give the impression to most of the people around them that they are still relatively unaware of how ill they are.

It would be an inexperienced and possibly insensitive doctor or nurse who assumed that the patient had no questions, no fears, no problems, because they did not articulate them. One of the highest skills to be developed in caring for the dying is that of heightened sensitivity and awareness — understanding what lies behind the comment or question, sensing the unspoken doubt or fear. The dying patient chooses his friends and confidants. He seeks information from one, comfort from another, reassurance from yet another, and denial from yet someone else. He expects each member of the primary care team to know as much about him and his future as all the others do, whether they are doctors or nurses. One morning he seems resigned to die and that same afternoon appears to be unaware of it and demonstrating sophisticated denial only to unburden himself of questions when the family doctor drops in after evening surgery.

His confidence and his courage may wax and wane as frequently and as painfully as at any other time of life. The least thing can upset that balance. It only needs a casual remark by doctor or nurse to undo much that the team has done. One hint that they are too tired to listen, too busy to stay longer, one glance at their watch, and an opportunity may have been lost to them never to return.

With the dying every remark, every expression of the face may have significance. Every moment is precious and no one is more conscious of time than the man or woman facing death. It is a myth that caring for the dying needs time which every doctor and nurse will agree is hard to find. The dying do not ask much time of us — they do ask that the time spent with them be devoted entirely to them, and that no impression ever be left with them that they are in any way of lesser importance, lesser priority, than those who can be cured.

They do not value trite platitudes any more than they expect false hopes. They look for honesty even when the most honest answer may be 'I don't know'. They lose their fear and come to face the future when they find in their doctors and nurses people courageous and compassionate enough to walk with them those last few miles as caring companions rather than as highly trained professionals. There are not, there can never be, rules about communicating with the dying, except perhaps one. We should communicate with them in word, deed and expression as we would have people deal with us. We all respond to love and respect, to honesty and dignity, to physical contact and human companionship. The dying are that one stage further along the road of life than we are, and know and sense this even more than we do. Giving them these things is communicating.

7

Doctor–nurse co-operation

It is no exaggeration to say that good domiciliary terminal care is not possible without co-operation between the general practitioner and community nurse. This chapter will look at what is meant by co-operation and how it may be achieved.

Of course patients may die at home without a community nurse ever having been involved. The death may have been sudden and unexpected as a result of myocardial infarction or cerebral vascular catastrophe but such patients cannot really be said to have been in need of terminal care if their illness was so short and the death so sudden. Others again, it must be recognized, refuse to have community nurses involved in their care because they preferred to be looked after by relatives, wanted to be independent, or were just obstinate and 'difficult'!

Sadly, however, some spend their last months at home, or even die there, without any professional nurses attending to them because the doctor failed to call in these colleagues. Others have nurses in attendance but they are involved too late to prevent pressure sores, or the co-operation between doctor and nurse is so poor that less than optimum benefit follows their involvement. The blame may lie with the doctor or the nurse or with both. Such patients suffer and what has been provided cannot possibly be described as 'good terminal care'.

The professional skills and role of the family doctor are well recognized by patients, families and nursing colleagues. Usually their inadequacies are equally recognized even if not spoken of. The skills of community nurses are less well recognized by many family doctors and even by some families.

By her basic and post-registration training, and subsequent experience, she is qualified to:

1. Provide, and advise on, all aspects of practical nursing;
2. Advise on dietary regimes;
3. Advise on aids which will facilitate caring and greater comfort;

4. Co-operate in family support;
5. Advise relatives on simple nursing procedures;
6. Interpret to patients and relatives some of the advice offered by her medical colleagues. (It is so often forgotten by doctors how little patients understand or retain what doctors explain to them and how much more approachable and acceptable the nurse may be.)
7. Prepare patients for admission to hospital or hospice;
8. Liaise with hospital nursing colleagues;
9. Obtain equipment and nursing aids for use in the home;
10. Arrange for night-sitters or Marie Curie nurses.

Like all good professionals involved in providing terminal care, the community nurse should aim to anticipate problems rather than correct or improve what has already happened. She can only do this if she is given the opportunity and the encouragement. The only way that this can happen is for her to be involved at the earliest possible stage and, for this, she requires co-operation from her medical colleagues.

Problems arise for some of the following reasons.

1. The doctors and nurses do not meet regularly and frequently enough as a team in the practice. If there is, for example, a weekly meeting, the patient whose condition is recognized as entering the terminal phase will be mentioned and the nurse can offer either to start visiting, *or* ask in which way she can help *or* ask that the doctor keep her informed about the patient so that she can become involved as soon as it is thought her help would be useful.

2. The doctor does not appreciate all the nurse might be able to do, even by way of advice without practical nursing, at an early stage. Even when a patient is still ambulant she can advise on walking aids, commodes, back-rests, urinals, sheepskins, diet etc.

3. The nurse, already involved, fails in her responsibility to plan her care programme. She continues to visit weekly when more frequent visits are obviously necessary. She fails to see what aids will assist or what additional support and guidance for the relatives might achieve. Once invited into the care of a patient it is *her* responsibility to decide how often she should visit, what she should do, and what additional nursing help should be invoked. The doctor's responsibility in this respect ended when the nurse was called in.

4. The nurse may let the patient and doctor down by failing to observe and report every single problem which calls for medical

help and intervention. She allows the patient to report pain, insomnia, sweating, nausea or dyspnoea and does not immediately contact the doctor. She fails to check for oral thrush, fails to advise on oral hygiene, fails to check on bowel evacuation, colostomy-functioning, or neglects to report to the doctor on new fears expressed by the patient or family.

5. The doctor fails his patient and nursing colleague by not displaying due professional respect for her skills and competence. She reports that the patient has thrush but he either doubts her diagnostic skills, leaves it until his next week's visit to confirm it, or refuses to prescribe nystatin for immediate assistance. Her anxieties about inadequate ostomy appliances are not met by either a visit or an invitation to the local stoma sister. Her mentioning of poor pain control is countered with the observation that 'He seemed okay when I was in!' or a less than polite reminder that prescribing is the doctor's domain!

6. Either the doctor or nurse, sometimes both, may be uncomfortable caring for the dying. They focus on physical problems to the exclusion of the many emotional, social or spiritual problems. They studiously avoid spending long with the patient, go to any lengths to avoid eye contact, tend to 'pass the buck' to the other ('You will have to speak to Sister about that' or 'Why didn't Doctor do anything about that?')!

Such observations may, to some readers, seem so foreign that they cannot believe they ever happen. They are based on the observations by the author over many years and confirmed by medical and nursing colleagues across the country. Few of us are comfortable with the dying, few are skilled in terminal care, and all of us have failed in one way or another on many occasions. All can improve and look afresh at how we co-operate with each other. The following suggestions may help.

1. Hold regular meetings of the primary care team or, if there is no attached community nurse, set regular times aside for meetings between doctor and nurse.

2. Each doctor with a terminally ill patient under his care should mention him or her at each meeting, giving the following information:

   a. The current state of his health and the progression of the disease. (The nurse needs to know this every bit as much as the doctor.)

   b. Details of current problems and how the doctor plans to manage them—drugs, aids, equipment, psychological support, information given to the patient, time with relatives etc.

c. Details of investigations, hospital reports, clinic follow-up, and future plans. The nurse needs to know if readmission is planned, chemotherapy or radiotherapy envisaged, the help of a Pain Relief Clinic being sought etc.

d. Areas in which doctor and nurse may co-operate. The nurse is thus encouraged and entitled to report on her work, what she plans, changes she has witnessed and what help she hopes for from the doctor.

3. Arrangements must be made for 'ad hoc' meetings or contacts between doctor and nurse as the intensity of care increases. It may be daily before morning surgery, each morning over coffee, or at the end of the day by telephone.

4. By prior arrangement the doctor and nurse should occasionally visit the patient together so that they may be seen to work as a partnership and be seen to agree and support each other.

5. Each doctor must be responsible for ensuring that his medical colleagues and any who deputize for him are fully conversant with every relevant detail of the care programme. There can *never* be an excuse for a nurse attending a dying patient at the weekend finding herself turning for help to a doctor who knows nothing about that patient.

6. Each nurse must ensure that her nursing colleagues know all they need to about the patient when she is on 'days off'. Optimally, this will be achieved by a few minutes of conversation but much good can still follow the leaving of a concise, precise report in a sealed envelope in the patient's house.

7. Doctor and nurse must be seen and heard to be saying the same thing! Nothing is more damaging and upsetting for the patient than for a nurse not to know or understand why a particular drug is being given or for a doctor to visit and not be sure why Sister has said this or that.

Dying patients, whether they look it or not, are usually frightened and insecure. Anything which suggests to them that professional attendants are not in control of the situation will make them worse, their pain more severe, their hope fade, or their request for readmission to hospital more pressing and persuasive.

8

Co-operating with hospitals, hospices and clinics

Approximately 90% of the last year of life is usually spent at home under the care of the family doctor and community nurses. Admissions to hospital are usually for courses of radiotherapy and chemotherapy, the treatment of intercurrent infections, constipation or sub-acute obstruction, or to provide a respite for the relatives. To colleagues working in hospital such admissions, particularly for cancer patients, seem so frequent that it is easy for them to forget how much care is being given to the patient at home. It is equally easy for members of the primary care team to forget how much they know and are always learning about the patient and fail to keep hospital colleagues updated. The result, sadly, is sometimes less co-operation and mutual respect than are required and the patient and family becoming increasingly aware of these poor communications.

The following guidelines are suggested to improve this most essential co-operation.

HOSPITALS

Correspondence

All referral letters should include the following information:
1. An up-to-date diagnosis (including complications).
2. A detailed list of current medication, including the times when drugs have been taken.
3. The results of any recent investigations, with dates.
4. The patient's knowledge of the condition and its seriousness with any relevant remarks made or questions that have been asked.
5. A brief description of how the condition and complications have been described by the members of the primary care team.
6. Any relevant information about the social circumstances in-

cluding health and 'coping' in family members and problems they have raised.

7. Details of ways in which the primary care team hope to co-operate in the future, including follow-up, treatment monitoring, frequency of domiciliary nursing that is possible, and which general practitioner partner can be contacted for discussion.

Some of these points merit expansion.

Though the primary diagnosis may well be known to hospital colleagues if the patient has been in their unit in the past, they need to know of recent infections (and treatment), new neurological features, recent cardiac failure, newly proven or suspected malignant metastases, and any newly recognized allergies.

Nothing is more upsetting for a patient than for a hospital doctor to be asking what medication they are on, or putting them back on to an antibiotic, diuretic, analgesic or laxative, which has been tried at home and found ineffective.

Sadly many hospitals seem to ignore the results of investigations organized by general practitioners and repeat everything, often at considerable expense and unnecessary upset to the patient. The family doctor is not responsible for changing hospital routine but he can help by giving all the information he has.

Even more important is that all concerned in the care should appear to say the same thing! If the family doctor has been able to guide the patient to an understanding of his condition (possibly after weeks of patient home visiting) it is to be hoped that the information he shares with the hospital would enable the hospital doctors and nurses to build on that. It is, for example, so helpful to report that the patient undoubtedly knows how serious it is and has even talked freely and at length about it, yet still speaks to relative strangers as though he had no insight whatsoever. His 'denial' can easily be understood and respected without anyone having to create confusion by telling him outright lies.

No one in hospital is ever likely to be as aware of all the social details of a patient as a family doctor particularly if, as is so often the case, he looks after other family members. For the hospital to be informed that the husband is, on the whole, managing well but has recently resorted to higher alcohol intake or that the domestic situation will improve when his wife's sister comes to help them, could be very helpful.

Unfortunately hospital staff do not always know details of local practices, whether there are attached community nurses, how frequently they could visit, whether a deputizing service is employed etc. They can be helped by being told of this, whether the family doctor will do follow-up blood tests, whether he wants the patient to return to the hospital out-patient department, whether he wants to be present when information about discharge is given to the patient in the hospital and whether he himself wants to be the one to 'tell'.

Personal contact

Make personal contact (whether as a doctor or nurse) with the opposite number in hospital. There is no reason why the family doctor should not arrange to speak to his consultant colleague at a mutually convenient time, either by visiting the hospital or by telephone. Likewise the community nurse can, if it is geographically possible, visit the ward sister or telephone to get and give all the necessary information when a patient is admitted and again prior to discharge. It is so heartening for a patient to hear his doctor say that, 'As I was saying to Dr . . . . only yesterday when we talked about you . . .' 'Yes, Sister . . . . . . told me how the new dressings had helped so we will continue with them at home'.

Define professional responsibilities and objectives

This is particularly relevant for doctors and has, to some extent, been alluded to already. It is not suggested that the family doctor try to teach his hospital colleagues nor dictate to them. It does help all concerned, and not least the patient whose needs and feelings should be central, if each knows what the other is thinking and planning. Some examples might illustrate this point.

If the family doctor sends the patient to hospital for tapping of a pleural effusion, it helps if he explains that as soon as that has been done and he is more comfortable the doctor is eager to have him home, no matter how ill he is. If he refers a patient as much so that a colleague can repeat explanations and reassurances that have already been given but not understood or accepted, this must be said.

Many very ill patients waste precious energy and time by repeated follow-up visits to clinics when it is well recognized by all concerned that no new treatment will result. They are being called back because different consultants, with kind and thoughtful intentions, did not want the patient to feel he had been forgotten. (It would have to be admitted that sometimes it is for completeness of statistics, experience for junior staff in training, or because no one thought to discontinue inappropriate follow-up.) It is the right of a family doctor in these circumstances to get in touch with the consultant concerned and ask if such out-patient visits are really necessary, explaining what he himself is prepared and able to do, and reassuring that copies of letters to colleagues will continue to be sent for completeness of records. There seems little point in a lady with carcinoma of breast being followed up by a surgical team who did a mastectomy five years before when she is already attending a radiotherapist, medical oncologist, and possibly a Pain Clinic. This is an example of the potential benefits of Combined Clinics.

Is it necessary for a patient on cytotoxics to be taken to a hospital clinic for a blood count when it can be done by the family doctor and a copy be sent by the laboratory to the oncologist? Need a patient return to hospital for cathether change or bladder lavage when community nurses are more than capable of doing this?

Maintain contact with the patient in hospital

Admittedly this may be a counsel of perfection in some areas where specialist hospitals are so far away from the patient's home and the base of the primary care team but in many towns and cities it can be done. Even one hospital visit lasting less than five minutes can do more to cheer a patient than any drugs. It also puts a face to the name of the family doctor for hospital staff, gives them a minute to share some details of the patient's problems and shows the patient how all are working together.

HOSPICES

For brevity this term is here used to describe hospices (independent and NHS), Continuing Care Units, Marie Curie Foundation Homes and Sue Ryder Homes. They are now to be found all over the country, some as small as five-bedded units and others with sixty or more beds. The larger ones have full-time medical staff of both consultant and junior grade, whilst others are served by local practitioners. All aspire to a high nurse:patient staff ratio and may have physioterapists, occupational therapists, social workers, chaplains and many volunteers, helping to create an atmosphere which is homely and relaxed whilst, at the same time, losing nothing of the professional excellence which has made some of the British ones world-famous.

They all care for patients with far-advanced disease, though only maligant disease in the case of the Marie Curie Memorial Foundation Homes, and some are prepared to admit for holiday respite. The emphasis is on quality of living rather than preparation for dying with most laying stress on pain and symptom palliation and, where possible, rehabilitation home for a time.

It is impossible to give hard and fast rules about co-operation with them because each unit functions slightly differently. It is therefore the responsibility of the family doctor to get to know the policy of his nearest unit, and if possible the colleagues there, so as to make best use of the facilities.

The points he needs to know are as follows.

Referral procedures

1. Are there forms to be completed?
2. Is there a waiting list or some other system of allocating priorities?
3. Is a pre-admission assessment visit done by a hospice doctor?
4. Are non-cancer patients accepted?

Stage of illness for eligibility

Some hospices only accept those dying in the near future whilst others are primarily palliative care units willing and keen to accept patients with many weeks or months of life, suffering pain or other symptoms proving difficult to control at home.

Perception and knowledge of the diagnosis

It is probably true to say that no hospice requests or requires that the patient first be 'told' he is suffering from far-advanced illness before he is accepted. Nevertheless this matter often troubles doctors who feel that admission to a hospice will be regarded as a death sentence by the still optimistic patient. This is also a cause of anxiety for relatives who have determinedly protected the patient from the truth and now, whether they admit it or not, dread being faced by a loved one who never suspected and now blames them for having told him lies. As is described elsewhere in this book, this is very rarely the case – most patients have deduced the state of their illness even if they have not explicitly been told and are usually very relieved to be in a unit so capable of controlling suffering and yet so friendly and understanding.

The family doctor nevertheless obviously has to make a delicate and sometimes difficult decision when he refers a patient to a hospice. The better he knows both the unit and his medical colleagues there, the easier it will be for him and all concerned.

Is there an out-patient department or Day Hospice?

It makes contact with the unit much easier if a patient can be seen initially at an out-patient department or, if the hospice has one, can attend a Day Hospice or Day Centre.

Experience shows that it is very rare indeed for a patient or relative to continue with their impression of the local hospice as a 'death house' or place of 'doom and gloom' when they have been seen as an out-patient or attended a Day Hospice.

Is there an associated Macmillan Service?

Throughout Britain there are now hundreds of Macmillan nurses so named because the initial funding for each Service comes from the Macmillan Fund of the National Society for Cancer Relief whose founder was Douglas Macmillan. A few are employed by hospices, the remainder by Health Boards.

Each nurse is an experienced Nursing Sister, qualified in community nursing, probably with experience as a health visitor, who has done further courses in terminal care nursing and other associated subjects such as oncology, counselling and ostomy care.

Macmillan nurses are not substitutes for community nurses but work alongside them and other members of the primary care team to bring additional expertise in pain and symptom control, family support, grief counselling, and improve liaison with specialist clinics and colleagues. They are capable, provided the members of the primary care team enable and encourage them to do so, to bring to domiciliary care all that is good in hospice care and can make all the difference to the support of both patient and family.

Some Macmillan nurses work alone whilst others are backed up by hospice physicians who may share in the initial visit when the Service is called in by the family doctor and then remain available to help with any new problems or difficulties which might arise.

Like any professional service, a Macmillan one is only as good as the people who staff it and co-operate with it.

PAIN RELIEF CLINICS

Though increasing in number with a much increased interest in pain control particularly amongst anaesthetists, there are still not sufficient clinics for the whole country. It is the responsibility of the family doctor to know where the nearest clinic is, its mode of referral, the services it offers and the colleagues who operate it. As always, personal contact makes all the difference.

Most clinics are directed by consultant anaesthetists or hospice physicians, supported by junior medical staff, radiographers, physiotherapists, and often with attending clinical psychologists.

They are equipped to carry out sophisticated 'nerve block' procedures (on an out-patient or in-patient basis), provide TENS (trans-cutaneous electrical nerve stimulators), hypnotherapy, biofeedback, relaxation, acupuncture, and advise on pharamacological methods of pain control. It is sometimes wrongly thought that they employ only physical or non-drug methods but in fact many of their successes follow on the skilled prescribing of appropriate analgesic drugs, sometimes supplemented where possible by physical methods. The availability of a clinical psychologist is a reminder that they regard pain as affecting, and being affected by, the whole person.

Inevitably many patients referred to such pain relief clinics are suffering from apparently intractable pain from benign pathologies where the doctor has tried everything known to him without success. Often a major psychological overlay, or personality disorder, are found to be important factors in the problem, as the family doctor had long recognized.

Patients with far-advanced progressive disease who might benefit from referral might include those with pancreatic carcinoma, perineal recurrence of a rectal carcinoma (in whom a coeliac plexus block might be considered), those with hepatic or intrathoracic pain (a para-vertebral block), those with ENT tumours susceptible to various neurolytic procedures, intrapelvic pain, unilateral pain (possibly benefiting from percutaneous cordotomy), post-herpetic neuralgia and many others.

Vitally important is that the doctor send the most detailed referring letter describing the problems, the pain, the many medications tried, and his own assessment of the patient's personality and social relationships. Ideally he should not regard the pain relief clinic as a last resort when all else has failed.

THE CLINICAL PSYCHOLOGIST

It is well recognized that many general practitioners never have the benefit of a clinical psychologist to assist with their patients in a whole professional lifetime. When they are fortunate enough to have access they should ascertain how to refer patients and what particular skills the local psychologist has to offer.

In addition to the help they may bring to those with hysterical and personality affected conditions, enuresis, behavioural disorders, asthma, allergies and the like, they have a major role to play in the care of the terminally ill.

Often it is found that pain does not respond to what would seem to be appropriate analgesic regimes with due attention to pain threshold, the environment and full support of patient and family. The question must then be asked if there is an underlying personality problem. Does the patient have to have pain to command sympathy or attention? Is he one of those who sees pain as a 'cross to bear', a punishment? Is there a hysterical element? Is his response to pain a manipulative technique? In these and similar cases the assessment and advice of a clinical psychologist can be invaluable.

Referring may not be easy! 'So you are saying it is all in my mind doctor!' 'You don't really think I am imagining this hell do you?' The last thing the doctor wants is to antagonize a patient particularly when months of terminal care lie ahead, but equally the doctor can see that no amount of drugs will achieve all he would like. It is often easier to explain that the psychologist is an expert at helping the person to cope better with his pain and suffering, able to show him skills and strengths within himself which he never knew he had. At all costs the doctor must avoid giving the impression that he believes the pain is in the patient's 'imagination' or made worse because he is 'neurotic' or a coward.

After all the pain *is* real, *is* unbearable to the patient. We are hoping to bring him to a better understanding of it, of himself, and of his ability to combat it or live with it.

9

Spiritual needs

It may be tempting for the doctor or nurse to ignore the spiritual needs of the dying patient. They may assume that the local or family clergyman will cope with the problems, forgetting that fewer and fewer people have Church connections and many 'non-attenders' may not be known to the parish priest or minister. For an unknown clergyman to be called in to help (with the patient's permission) must be as daunting for him as for a deputizing doctor visiting a strange patient.

A more common reason for not becoming involved in spiritual questions is that faith is a very personal matter and a doctor must not ever be seen as imposing his own beliefs on a patient or family. Coupled with this fear might be the fact that many doctors and nurses have not felt the need for a living faith and feel unqualified to help others in spiritual need. They feel ill-equipped to answer questions which they may never have encountered or raised in their own lives.

It does seem however that close on three-quarters of dying patients raise spiritual issues in their final weeks of life. No matter how 'non-religious' or 'non-practising' they may have been in times of health, they now feel a need to question the presence of God, the love and forgiveness of God, the possibility of an after-life and reunion with loved ones (and also those they have not loved) and their need to pray. Some, far from seeking the comfort of faith, feel compelled to blame God for apparently being so callous, so unfair or so vindictive. They see their illness and approaching death ·as proof of His failure to answer prayers and His indifference to mortal man.

It is not expected of any doctor or nurse that they should know all the answers any more than they should know everything there is to be known of medicine and its many specialties. Each patient does, however, have the right to expect and hope that his doctor or nurse will see his needs, hear his spoken or unspoken cries for help, and at least either listen or know where to turn for 'specialist' help. In the same way that no doctor would turn a deaf ear to a social problem which is affecting his patient's health he cannot turn away from spiritual ones no matter how daunting they may seem.

The family doctor, of all the many professionals involved in the care of someone with far-advanced disease, is best placed to uncover problems and either solve them himself or find someone qualified to do so. In good practice the boundaries between physical, emotional, social and spiritual are so blurred as to be of no consequence whatsoever.

GUIDELINES FOR ASSISTING WITH SPIRITUAL PROBLEMS

1. As early as possible in the care of such a patient ascertain if there is a Church connection and whether or not there is regular, though not necessarily frequent, contact with a clergyman.

2. At an appropriate time ask if the minister or priest is aware of the patient's state of health and whether the patient would like the doctor to have a word with him. It is usually easy to reassure that just as the doctor is trained to respect confidentiality and will only pass on information with the patient's consent and if it might assist the minister to help more, so also is the minister someone who respects confidentiality.

3. If contact can be made in this way then develop co-operation with the minister by explaining the 'medical' care and objectives and then suggesting ways in which the clergyman might be able to assist the members of the primary care team as well as the patient. Many doctors give clergy the impression that they have no role, no contribution, when in fact they often have knowledge of relationships, past crises and coping, and personalities which complement the knowledge of the doctor. Just as doctors have until recently had little or no specific training in terminal care and bereavement counselling, so has the preparation for the ministry often been lacking. Ministers are often acutely aware of this and feel both daunted by the challenge and excluded by doctors whom society have elected to 'manage' death. Their training too is improving and many have profound skills in personality assessment, family dynamics and counselling techniques.

4. Do not fall into the trap of trying to answer the spiritual and philosophical questions and observations of the patient. When someone asks why God does something, or what God is thinking

about, much as he might like to know the answer, he is not likely to expect even his trusted family doctor or nurse to know the Mind of God!

5. Do not offer trite platitudes! In all probability, nothing which is said at this time by way of explanation, no matter how well intentioned, is likely to comfort. 'Don't worry about all you've done—I am sure God understands!' may not reassure someone terrified of damnation.

6. If the doctor or nurse has a personal faith, they need not expand on it (tempting as that may be) but just showing that they have one can be of inestimable help—even by admitting that they too have many unanswered questions. The dying often feel they should be clear about everything when all that is happening is bewildering and seems to make no sense. To be cared for by someone who also has questions and even doubts but still believes, can still be helpful. 'I am like you—I simply don't know why this happens—but I am still very sure there is a God who cares and who can forgive'.

7. Be particularly sensitive to the believing person who has always found comfort in prayer and now, like so many desperately ill people, finds it almost impossible to pray or even be confident that God is listening. Such people are often more upset by what they see as a lapse of faith or a distancing from God than by any other features of their illness or dying. Even being reassured that most people experience this difficulty in praying can be a comfort.

8. Respect beliefs and customs which seem in conflict with professional medical knowledge. The fact that we have no explanation for any effectiveness of anointing with oil or taking Holy Water should not affect our attitude or our care.

9. Do not be dismayed by the patient praying for a cure—it does not necessarily mean they expect it or have not understood and accepted the doctor's explanation and now need a longer and more detailed explanation.

10. Be prepared to help the relatives who are perplexed by the patient who turns to God after a lifetime of rejecting or denying Him. Many dying patients find Him at the end, just at the same time that their relatives may be losing any faith they ever had. God becomes more real to the dying when He becomes more inexplicable than ever to the living.

11. If it is possible, meet with the clergyman at the bedside to demonstrate both mutual respect and shared caring for all the needs of the patient.

DIFFERENT FAITHS AND CULTURES

In areas where there are many different ethnic communities, the doctor and nurse may easily be baffled by differing beliefs and customs and anxious lest they inadvertently say or do the wrong thing.

Some of the basic facts of these faiths and cultures as they relate to dying are given below as guidelines for all concerned. Only the most general principles are given.

Buddhists

The time between death and committal depends on the lunar calendar and varies from three to seven days. The most important thing is for the Buddhist Priest to be informed as soon as possible and most Buddhists will be ready to provide the name of one of the same school of Buddhism as the deceased. If possible the body should not be moved before the priest arrives to say the necessary prayers though they can be recited at a distance, in a Temple for example.

Chinese

On the death of a child the burial takes place at once with no special ceremony after the body has been washed.

With adults, the body is washed and then, if tradition is followed, clothed in white after which the bedding that has been prepared for the coffin is put on the bed and the body laid on it so that relatives and friends may see the body before it is placed in the coffin.

Hindus

It has to be remembered that Hindus are strict vegetarians though some, but by no means all, will eat eggs and dairy produce which is free of animal fat. Strict Hindus will not eat even vegetarian items if they have been cooked near, or served with, utensils used for meats of any kind.

When a Hindu is dying, relatives may wish to bring money and clothes for him to touch before distribution to the needy. Some will ask to sit at the bedside and read from a Holy book.

After the death, the relatives will wash the body, preferably in running water, and put on new clothes. Some Temples have special facilities for this and occasionally arrangements can be made with hospital mortuaries for the body to be washed by relatives on the post-mortem tables as water is run over it. If a post-mortem has to be performed they will be anxious for all organs to be returned to them before the mandatory cremation which will usually be arranged for the earliest possible time.

Jews

Jews have strict dietary customs which they are happy to explain to non-Jewish doctors and nurses attending them.

After death the burial (cremation is forbidden) usually takes place within 24 hours, the body being prepared by someone of the same sex with three members of the community in attendance. A male member of the family may remain with the body until the funeral and seven days of strict family mourning observed afterwards.

Muslims

Lamb, beef, goat, chicken and rabbit are allowed if they have been killed by a Muslim with a religious prayer (Halal). Pork, carrion and blood are forbidden as are all forms of alcohol. Fish and eggs are allowed but cannot be cooked where any of the forbidden meats have been.

After the death, the body must not be touched by a non-Muslim. Unless it is required by law, a post-mortem should not be requested. The body is washed by the family and no coffin is used.

Sikhs

Sikhs do not eat beef and some Sikh women do not eat meat of any kind.

After death, as for the Hindus, the body must be washed in running water by the relatives and then be cremated as soon as possible.

10

Bereavement

With his commitment to continuing care of a family, the family doctor is better placed than any other professional, including his nursing colleagues or the clergy, to provide skilled, compassionate bereavement support. He is the one to whom the patient and probably many of the close relatives will first come when a sinister diagnosis is suspected, then confirmed; the one who will monitor the progress of the condition, often over many years, until death occurs; the one who has the privilege of providing terminal care at home and continuing his care of the family for years to come.

This does not imply that the community nurse has no role in preparing for bereavement or mitigating its impact but her involvement with the family, usually so intense whilst she provides the terminal nursing care, often ceases after the death. The social worker may be better placed than even doctor or nurse but few practices have them in the team, most have sadly to place lower priority on bereavement than they would wish, and seldom are they involved with many of the families who lose a loved one at home. The clergy should be key carers in this area but fewer and fewer families have close Church connections and, like some doctors, there are members of the clergy who, whilst meaning well, have little knowledge of the many facets and faces of grief.

GRIEF

There are some things about grief which, though apparently self-evident, bear repeating.

Grief starts when the diagnosis is made

Particularly is this the case with cancer, even though a relatively good prognosis is given for the next few years. Worse is the case of the patient who is not informed of the diagnosis or prognosis (often at the request of well-meaning relatives) and the family then add to the sadness in their own lives the burden of 'conspiracy of silence'.

Each relapse is a reminder of further loss and what is still to come. Each new symptom adds to their suffering and pain. Nothing could be more dangerous or detrimental than for the members of the primary care team to focus all attention on the patient until he dies, leaving the family to grieve unnoticed or unaided.

Grief is not always physiological

Sadly there are still many doctors and nurses who make little or no attempt to help the grievers because 'sadness is a natural emotion'. One can palliate grief as much as one can palliate the suffering of the dying. The professional who leaves them to grieve unsupported, before or after the death, is usually betraying his own sense of inadequacy.

Grief can be predicted

Some guidelines to assist in prediction and preparation will be given in this chapter. At the very least, the doctor can acknowledge with the family that he recognizes something of what they are suffering, whether it is sadness, guilt, failure or even relief.

Grief carries a definite morbidity

Even if a doctor chooses not to provide planned support, he has a responsibility to remember the morbidity attached to grief, particularly in widowers, and set out to practise preventive care by appropriate follow-up.

Grief may change families beyond recognition

So dramatic, and sometimes so drastic, are the changes wrought by a death in the family, the doctor has a responsibility to be on the alert for its effects on every single family member on his list, whether it be the adolescent or the old widow, the chronic neurotic or the alcoholic. No family is ever the same again, for better or worse, after a death. Beyond question there are some families who are better after a death than they were before. The young, rebellious teenager seems to mature overnight. The wayward, pleasure-seeking daughter takes on new domestic responsibilities. The browbeaten wife enjoys a happiness and freedom she has never known before. With skill, it is possible for the different members of the primary care team to capitalize on the potential of many family members and, paradoxical as it may sound, bring good out of sadness and tragedy.

Factors affecting grief outcome

1. Time to prepare for the deceased's death.
2. Griever's sense of usefulness in caring for the deceased.
3. Griever's perception of personal support received.
4. Previous personality.
5. Quality of relationship with the deceased.

Sudden, unexpected death, produces the profoundest emotional shock and subsequent grief reaction whereas time spent caring for the dying patient, whether he had cancer or any other pathology, will often lessen the reaction. This book is primarily about 'prolonged dying' rather than sudden, unexpected death. Nevertheless it is worth reiterating here that every immediate relative of someone dying unexpectedly must be regarded as 'at risk' and their primary care team plan accordingly.

It is certainly not true that the longer a carer nurses a dying patient the less is the grief. Throughout much of that time, the carer, like the patient himself, may subconsciously deny the diagnosis and sinister prognosis. At other times he or she may be acutely aware of the outcome when the patient goes into a relapse, particularly with cancer. However, just when they feel prepared for the inevitable death, the patient enters a remission as a result of further radiotherapy, chemotherapy or surgery. This ebb and flow of grief can be particularly traumatic for the loving relative as much as it may elevate and depress the mood of the patient. Frequently there comes a time when the relative feels they can take no more, yet the patient is enjoying a remission. Inevitably there is guilt, embarrassment and shame, and this period of 'wishing he was dead' is alluded to after the death. It is important that each member of the primary care team recognizes the strain imposed on relatives who, though very willing to nurse the patient and do all possible for him, nevertheless are traumatized by the frequent relapses and remissions so common under modern treatment regimes.

The more 'useful' a relative can be made to feel, the less will be the grief. The modern tendency to hospitalize most seriously ill and dying patients in the mistaken belief that they need such facilities and that most relatives are unwilling and unable to care for them at home, has important implications for the grievers who may thus be deprived of an opportunity to demonstrate their love and devotion to the patient. Each member of the primary care team has a responsibility to encourage and enable relatives to do as much nursing as possible, both for the immediate benefit of the patient and for the later effect on the griever's own reaction. There are few people who cannot be taught bed-bathing, sponging, oral hygiene, appropriate positioning in bed, feeding techniques, the preparation of appetizing meals, the completion of pain charts etc. Every family doctor can recall relatives who were later troubled by guilt in case their loved one had been taken to hospital, not for specialist nursing but because the family were inadequate or failing in some way or other. Even when this is perhaps the case, the family doctor should always explain that he is recommending hospital or hospice admission where there are 'more hands to help' or 'more people there at night' or 'doctors available at a minute's notice' — anything to prevent worsening of the guilt reaction.

Several studies have shown that the griever's perception of the support given to them is more important that the amount of support actually given. Some insight into their perception of support is probably more easily ascertained by a Health Visitor or clergyman than by the general practitioner or community nurse and obviously may be related to the previous personality and relationship with the deceased. As a useful rule of thumb, the griever who seems unaware of, and certainly unappreciative of, the many visits by the doctor, clergyman, kindly neighbours and many others, is certainly at risk.

Contrary to what might be expected, patients with extrovert personalities usually suffer the worse reactive depression but, predictably, those with dependent personalities who had leaned heavily on the one they have now lost, will intuitively seek someone else on whom to depend. These are features of which a general practitioner should already be aware, and for which he should be able to prepare. The person with an inflexible, obsessional personality will find adapting to a new way of life especially difficult and carers have to appreciate that most people cope with grief in the same way that they have coped with any other episodes of loss, whether of a job, status, or popularity. It is important to realize that intellectual prowess may bear no relationship to emotional maturity and stability.

Every family doctor has had the experience of encountering the most extreme demonstrations of grief in someone who has apparently been at loggerheads with the deceased as long as he can remember. He can look back on scores of consultations trying to reconcile the two, give them some better understanding of each other or even just to maintain a lukewarm marriage only to have the surviving one protest undying, unfathomable love, after he has gone. Equally there are those who even the longstanding family doctor had always thought were happily married and all in all to each other. After the death it transpires that the one who is left feels nothing but relief and freedom after what is said to have been a totally unhappy marriage.

Prediction of grief outcome

The following questions should be asked when preparing a plan of bereavement support or counselling by the primary care team.
1. Was the death expected and, if so, did it take the form expected by the bereaved?
2. Does the bereaved feel that he or she was enabled to do everything they wanted to do for the deceased and that what they did was appreciated by the patient and recognized by the professional attendants?
3. What is the personality type of the bereaved and what pattern of behaviour at a time of loss can be expected?
4. Have the bereaved be given adequate opportunity to ventilate even the most secret and unpleasant emotions they feel about the patient, his care, his attendants and themselves?

It is essential to appreciate that most, if not all, grievers will need to ventilate anger against some well-meaning medical or nursing colleague, God or even against the patient for being so inconsiderate to die as and when he did. It is equally important that the doctor does not defend, retaliate or attempt to rationalize, but instead he should permit an uninhibited outpouring. Some relatives may need to express relief or even happiness at the end of an unsatisfactory relationship but may feel unable to contravene the socially accepted grieving pattern.

Features of grief

More than 50% of bereaved people experience many of the symptoms suffered by the deceased during the first months after the loss, and understandably suspect that they are about to suffer a similar fate. This is particularly the case in cardiac and malignant disease with such symptoms as palpitations, breathlessness, chest tightness, weight loss, anorexia, dyspepsia and even dysphagia. In spite of their denial, and any professional confidence in the impact of health education, most lay people retain a sneaking fear than cancer is communicable.

The only way to deal with these symptoms, often reported with reluctance and embarrassment, is to conduct a single, thorough examination and the relevant investigations in as understanding a manner as possible, no matter how unlikely it is that anything organic will be found. Superficial, perfunctory or cursory examinations at the time of reporting of each new symptom will mean a heightening of anxiety or may encourage the fear of neuroticism and inadequacy. Unjustified as the feeling may be, many grieving relatives suspect that their loved one would still be alive if the diagnosis had been made more promptly or suspected earlier by the otherwise much-lived and respected family doctor. The 'knew' there was something seriously wrong when the doctor was treating him for bronchitis and only had him X-rayed after two weeks! They wondered why a barium meal was not ordered when he first reported his dyspepsia! They always felt that the doctor never took him seriously and were so grateful when the young trainee or locum spotted how serious it was! Such comments, common as they are, do not display a profound and lasting distrust in the family doctor. They do, however, make the patient that trifle more suspicious and less trusting when they themselves have something which requires investigation, or so they believe. The problem is compounded many times over when the family doctor has fallen into the trap of conspiring with them to tell lies to the dying patient. How are they to know if he is now being honest with them who found it so easy to persuade him that an untruth was preferable?

Ninety per cent of bereaved persons suffer disturbed sleep pattern in the first six months, with frequent wakening, with vivid dreams involving the deceased and bouts of profound misery (not to be confused with a true depressive state) at night. More than 50% will have auditory or visual hallucinations of the dead person, behaving exactly as he did in life. Fewer than 10% will report this for fear of being declared psychotic. On the other hand, many of these distresses will be reported freely to the health visitor. Patients describe how they reach over in bed and feel sure he is still lying beside them. They hear him put the milk bottles out at night in the way he has done for so many years, or stand at the kitchen door asking if she is ready to go to bed. They smell the loved one's pipe or the deceased wife's perfume. An explanation of these phenomena in advance re-inforcing that this is a normal aspect of bereavement saves much sadness and silent fear.

Totally unjustified as it may often be, almost all grief contains an element of guilt. Did they do enough, was it their fault, could they have coped longer at home, should they have encouraged more surgery or chemotherapy? Did he die because of that last tablet they gave? Was he crying on that final night because she had been impatient with him? The list is endless and the agony deep.

Stages of grief

Though seen in a more complete form after a protracted death as in cancer, respiratory or neurological disease, several 'stages' are seen in most grieving people. It would be quite wrong however to expect a steady progression from one stage to another or to hope that people would move through the stages as easily as they are described below. They are only described here as guidelines for the professional team.

It is generally accepted that there are five main stages in bereavement: (1) period of relief; (2) period of relaxing; (3) period of resenting; (4) period of remembering; (5) period of repairing.

Relief

This follows immediately on the death and usually lasts no more than days. It is characterized by happiness for the deceased ('Thank goodness he will have no more suffering'), coupled with personal relief ('I couldn't have coped with much more' or 'I wouldn't have wanted him to be a cripple'). There is much expressed gratitude for the care-givers, especially for the family doctors and nurses and a pervading sense of unreality and numbness – 'I can't take it in' or 'I don't feel like crying'.

Visits by the doctor or health visitor may be appreciated at the time but are soon completely forgotten in this period of stunned insensibility. Hypnotics, usually demanded by relatives rather than by the remaining spouse, seldom if ever work but may be a token of the doctor's continuing role.

It cannot be emphasized strongly enough that patients may be very alarmed by their numbness and 'stupidity' at this time. Even their address can be forgotten, or telephone numbers of the family, the name of the family minister, and every word of advice that has recently been given by the professionals. On no account should the doctor or nurse embark on giving advice in any form at this time.

Relaxing

This follows the funeral and usually lasts only as long as near relatives remain with the widow or widower. This seems to be about three weeks at the most but creates a welcome sense of support and acceptance and shared pain. These weeks are usually filled with practical problems related to wills, possessions or insurance claims but the ready assistance and availability of family and minister prevent the impact of loneliness being felt until nearer the time for the relatives' departure. Nevertheless this is a time when precipitate decisions may be made about selling a house, emigrating or moving in with a daughter. Inappropriate advice is often given about these subjects or about getting rid of all visible reminders of the deceased. However, mementos such as photographs, letters and trophies, and many other personal, but very ordinary items should be kept and treasured for the time when the world, not the widow or widower, seems to have forgotten that the loved one ever existed.

This is a useful period in which the family doctor can visit around the time he knows the relatives will be departing. They will be reassured to know of his interest, glad to see him sitting with the grieving one, and able to reassure themselves of his continuing interest and care. His authoritative advice on not making precipitate decisions will carry great weight.

Resenting

This dates from the time of departure of the family and may last anything from three to four months coinciding, it will be noted, with the end of 'acceptable' grief in modern society. There is in this time a profound sense not only of loneliness but 'aloneness', of insecurity and self-pity, with much criticism both of self ('I should never have left him that night') and of professional helpers ('The doctor could have got here much sooner'). The expression of these feelings often takes the doctor and nurse by surprise. It seems such a short time to them since they were overwhelmed with expressions of gratitude. This is no time to rationalize or defend. It must be recognized that the grieving patient has vivid memories of the past and seems fearful of looking into a future without hope.

Their suffering is heightened by friends describing how well they look and by an increasing incidence of symptoms so similar to those experienced in the final illness by the deceased; symptoms that are not often mentioned to the doctor for fear of genuine pathology being found or of neurosis. The good outward appearance of health and coping leads to invitations to resume social and church activities. The pain however is felt not when in company but when returning to an empty house.

Business matters loom large, accounts have to be paid without advice from a spouse, and the commonest question asked is, 'How on earth will I cope?'. It is frequently reported by the grievers that the three months mark is noteworthy for the way friends and neighbours go out of their way to avoid casual meetings, crossing to the other side of the street rather than stopping to ask how she is. Particularly painful is the frequency with which people speak of their own happiness, their own planned holidays, and never once mention the name of the one who has died as if 'out of sight, out of mind'.

Remembering

This may start at three months and continue for at least another twelve or fifteen months with constant reminiscing and reliving of events before the death, coupled with a conscious effort to re-capture the happy emotions and experiences of the past. No longer is it quite so painful to speak of the death and seldom, unless it is becoming pathological or the patient has a personality disorder, is there much recrimination. Great efforts will be made to create only the happiest memories even if the marriage was not, in fact, a happy one. This is the time of the visual and auditory hallucina-tions already referred to and the time (around seven months) of most breakdowns and suicide attempts in those unable to face a future or cope with their guilt and aloneness.

This is a difficult time for the family doctor. The patient appears well, is frequently seen outside and all reports from colleagues and community suggest that he or she is recovering well. Naturally he will remain anxious about the person with a known personality disorder, or the one with a history of depressive illness. He will be alerted by the patient who continues to recall vividly all the unpleasant or recriminating minutiae of the final illness, without ever being able to see the kindness that was shown, the love that was given or the support that has been abundant ever since.

Repairing

The patient now begins to make a deliberate effort to make a fresh start, shown by positive and rational thinking and a careful appraisal of his or her resources and skills. New interests, hobbies and friendships are cultivated, and at each consultation with the family doctor some new evidence of this can usually be elicited. This is not to say that anniversaries, particularly birthdays, Christmas and the date of the death, are not extremely painful and often ignored completely by other family members and even by the doctor. It is a stage characterized by the expression 'life must go on'.

BEREAVEMENT SUPPORT BY THE DOCTOR

The following guidelines may assist.

1. Visit as soon after the death as possible, whether it took place at home or in hospital, to remind the patient of your continuing support and concern. This visit will probably be a short one, later forgotten by the patient but appreciated by relatives and certainly noted by neighbours. It is tempting at this visit to speak soothing words, offer trite platitudes or some attempt at words of comfort. Experience shows that seldom is anything which is said right in the mind of the griever. Deeply grateful as they may be for the professional attendance given, they are easily hurt by anything which is said, no matter how well intentioned. 'Now at last he is free from all his pain and suffering' is met with the 'I want him back'. The well-meant 'Now he is at peace with God' may be predictably met with 'Why couldn't God leave him with me?'. The rule for this visit should undoubtedly be 'the least said, the better'. It is the presence of the doctor as a token of respect and care rather than the words he uses, which will long remain in the memory of the family.

2. Visit again, and this time allocate sufficient time, at the time when the relatives plan to leave. Be positive in advice, emphatic in advising against precipitate action and reassuring about your concern for his or her own health. Do not succumb to the pleadings of the family that transquilizers or hypnotics be left 'in case she needs them'.

3. Book a visit or a consultation for three months and then conduct a careful, physical examination, giving the patient every opportunity to express deep fears and suppressed emotions. If necessary, be positive and ask specifically about the same symptoms which were experienced by the deceased. Take pains to explain the features of 'normal' grief because it is unlikely that anyone else will ever have explained them. Particularly, talk about the painful feelings of anger, the anguish of guilt, the sympathetic suffering with the deceased, the hallucinations already referred to, and the way in which the world seems to go on as if John or Mary had never existed.

4. Make an opportunity for a further consultation for six months later when the world accepts her 'everything is fine' but experience shows that the patient is now at most risk. It should not be left to the patient to make the appointment but be booked in advance and the receptionist advised to send a reminder in advance or the health visitor asked to drop in if the appointment is not kept. More relaxed and informal as it might sound, it is not as useful to visit the house as to have the patient at the surgery where the thorough examination may be carried out.

5. Keep a diary in the practice of dates of deaths of patients on your list for planned follow-up for the first year. Particularly useful, and usually much appreciated by the patient, is a short, informal visit to the house on the anniversary of the death. It will surprise the doctor to be told that he was probably the only one who seemed to remember that day. Many doctors are daunted by the prospect of keeping such a diary of dates, forgetting that not all their dead patients have left relatives on their list and the number who must be followed up is by no means unmanageable!

6. Make use of CRUSE or any other bereavement service in your area, no matter how enthusiastic are the members of the primary care team about bereavement support.

Grief is like a surgical wound, painful and ugly at first, gradually fading but still easily damaged and hurt, never disappearing and always a permanent reminder of profound pain, shock, change and fear.

Time does not heal—it only makes the scar less visible to onlookers!

PATHOLOGICAL GRIEF REACTIONS

It is very difficult to say when a physiological grief reaction has become a pathological one.

The following suggest abnormal grief reactions:

1. When grief occurs in someone known to have a serious personality disorder, history of severe depressive illness, or suicide attempts.
2. When the griever repeatedly speaks of suicide or persists with an attitude of utter hopelessness and low self esteem.
3. When the griever has no perception of support in spite of undoubted support being offered by professionals, friends and community.
4. When a griever appears to progress well in the first few months, taking up old interests and hobbies and remaking a social life only to regress and withdraw for no apparent reason. She stops attending Church and its other activities, declines invitations to social events, stops telephoning friends.
5. When visits become more frequent to the surgery for 'trivial' complaints, no serious organic cause is found, and all mental distress is denied.
6. When it is suspected that alcohol intake is increasing or the patient is taking tranquillizers or hypnotics not prescribed by the doctor.

No firm rules can be given on the management of such grief reactions. Untreated, they are not likely to improve spontaneously. They may progress to suicide or para-suicide, or to prolonged depressive illness and social isolation.

If the patient has had previous contact with a psychiatrist, this should be renewed as a matter or urgency. If the general practitioner feels that the management is within his professional capability, he must make due allowance for the time that it will take and advise all colleagues in the primary care team of his suspicions and his planned care regime. Only after prior discussion with officers of CRUSE and other bereavement support services, should such patients be referred to that service which may not be equipped for severe pathological grief, excellent as the counsellors are for all other clients.

PRESCRIBING IN BEREAVEMENT

Considerable pressures are often brought to bear on the doctor to prescribe antidepressants or hypnotics for the bereaved, not so much by the patient herself or himself as by well-meaning relatives. Failure or reluctance to do so is seen as uncaring or professional callousness but experience shows that such drugs will only help if used for the same strict clinical indications, and with the same caution, as at any other time. That is to say, hypnotics should be prescribed only when there is good evidence of a grossly disturbed sleep pattern, and even then in as low a dose as possible and for the shortest possible time. Antidepressants will be totally ineffective unless the classical features of a psychiatric depressive state are present. This is a time when, all too easily, a sedative-taking habit may be induced, the patient started on the long-term use of a tranquillizer such as diazepam, or a patient may turn to alcohol. It is the time when barbiturates seem to offer distinct advantages yet must be withheld at all costs.

If a sedative is thought desirable immediately after the death or when the family have dispersed leaving the griever alone and hopeless, it should be a benzodiazepine with a short half-life (e.g. lorazepam or temazepam) or dichloralphenazone. Nitrazepam is contraindicated because its long half-life produces mental blurring the next day and occasionally hallucinations.

When depressive features are present, it is useful to prescribe a sustained-release tricyclic, taken at night, such as amitriptyline or trimipramine. Repeat prescriptions must not be made available for any of these drugs without a consultation. This basic rule affords an excellent opportunity to see and support the patient in a way which is infinitely superior to any prescription. Strict instructions should be given that 'sleeping tablets' and 'tranquillizers' are not to be accepted from family or friends.

It cannot be stated strongly enough that, profoundly painful as bereavement is, its course is rarely altered by pharmacological means.

Appendix 1

DRUGS AND EQUIPMENT FOR THE DOCTOR'S BAG

The contents of any doctor's bag are very much a matter of personal preference and reflect his practice and possibly his personality. What follows is a list of drugs found useful in domiciliary terminal care, particularly for the emergencies already discussed.

Diamorphine 30 mg ampoules

Because most patients will be on opiate doses less than 30 mg diamorphine 4-hourly, this injectable opiate will usually suffice for such emergencies as haemorrhage, vertebral collapse, pathological fractures etc.

There is little to be said for combined preparations such as morphine with cyclyzine (Cyclimorph) where the opiate dose is so small that one does not need the anti-emetic with its propensity for producing sedation and confusion, particularly in the elderly.

Dexamethasone Injection (4 mg per ml in 2 ml amouples)

Reference has already been made to its usefulness in SVC obstruction, spinal cord compression, hypercalcaemia and acute cerebral oedema.

Hyoscine Hydrobromide (400 μg per ampoule)

This should be carried in readiness for the 'death rattle' which, though probably not apparent to the dying patient, is often the cause of much upset to the relatives. Often it is given after the rattle has already started when it cannot dry up secretions lying in the posterior oropharynx or trachea. Its optimum use is as a prophylactic but it must be remembered that it produces tachycardia which, in the semiconscious patient, may be alarming.

Rectal diazepam solution (Stesolid 10 mg per tube)

This is valuable for rapid sedation and tranquillization when the intravenous route is not thought necessary. For the young and those of small frame, 10 mg will suffice. For most adults 20 mg (2 tubes) will be found preferable, becoming effective within 15 minutes and lasting no longer than three hours.

Intravenous diazepam (Diazemuls 10 mg per ampoule)

Provided its respiratory depressant effect is remembered, this is a valuable, rapidly effective benzodiazepine, useful as a tranquillizer and anticonvulsant.

Intravenous lorazepam (Ativan)

It differs from diazepam in having a more marked amnesic effect and shorter half-life but can depress respiration.

Methotrimeprazine (Nozinan) Injections

This phenothiazine is valuable as a major tranquillizer, anti-emetic, antipruritic, anti-hiccups drug with a modest analgesic effect. It is however very sedating. It is useful in emergencies in an intra-muscular dose of 25–50 mg and can be repeated 4-hourly.

Urinary catheters and drainage bag

The size of catheters most commonly used are 14 and 16. A 2-litre drainage bag will usually suffice until a supply is obtained from a chemist or hospital.

It is presumed that the doctor will, as a routine, carry injectable forms of frusemide, metoclopramide and chlorpromazine.

Those with the requisite training and experience in its use may wish to carry 5 mg of 5% phenol in glycerine for emergency intercostal blocks for patients sustaining pathological rib fractures or, safer in domiciliary practice, a 20 ml bottle of 2% lignocaine for infiltration.

Appendix 2

USEFUL ADDRESSES

Each general practitioner and community nurse will know the address of local DHSS offices, community equipment store domiciliary physiotherapy and chiropody services, Social Work Department (and associated occupational therapy services) for their own area. Similarly they will know where oxygen may be obtained, which chemists are open at night and at weekends, and the routes of referral for hospital admission and urgent domiciliary consultations.

Below are listed further useful addresses where additional help may be obtained for the care of their terminally ill patients.

Hospices

An up-to-date list of all hospice-type units and services, their medical and nursing directors, number of beds and special facilities is obtainable from:

> Hospice Information Service
> 51/53 Lawrie Park Road
> Sydenham
> London
> SE26 6DZ

It should be noted that though most hospices specialize in the care of patients with far-advanced cancer most are prepared to admit patients with non-malignant disease, and some offer holiday admissions to give a respite to relatives.

National Society for Cancer Relief

This national charity has established and provided the initial funding for the many Macmillan Home Care Services in Britain, helped to build some of the NHS hospices, and is heavily committed to continuing education of the many professionals involved in terminal care units and services.

Equally important is its interest in providing financial assistance towards fuel bills, bus fares, extra linen or special foods and equipment (to list just a few common problems).

Application by the doctor, health visitor, community nursing sister or social worker should be made to:

> National Society for Cancer Relief
> Michael Sobell House
> 30 Dorset Square
> London
> NW1 6QL

Malcolm Sargent Cancer Fund

This cancer fund was established in 1968 to help children suffering from cancer, leukaemia and Hodgkin's disease. Financial help is available very quickly and may be used for anything which would relieve parents' anxieties or ease a child's time in hospital or at home. It ranges from help towards a treat for an ill child to assistance with heating bills or the costs of a final family holiday before a child dies. The address is:

> Malcolm Sargent Cancer Fund
> 6 Sydney Street
> London
> SW3 6PP

Pain Relief Clinics

These are now to be found in most major cities and, even when not formally listed as a local service, may be provided by one or more local anaesthetists to whom an enquiry or application may be sent.

The general practitioner wishing to refer to one in his area can obtain information from the local office of the Area Health Authority (England and Wales) or Regional Health Board (Scotland) or via the local hospice which, in some centres, operate their own clinics. Referral procedures vary, some taking patients on direct referral from general practitioners, others only via a hospital consultant.

CRUSE

This national charity exists to help people in their bereavement and offers skilled counsellors, social workers, group meetings, social events and very deep understanding of the process and the pain of grief.

Local branches are listed in the telephone directory or addresses may be obtained from the national headquarters:

> CRUSE
> CRUSE House
> 126 Sheen Road
> Richmond
> Surrey
> TW9 1UR

British Red Cross Society

In addition to its better known first aid and accident services, the Society operates stores of such useful equipment as commodes, wheelchairs, backrests, walking aids etc., available on loan.

The address will always be found in the telephone directory.

Marie Curie Memorial Foundation

In addition to its nursing and sitter services operated by the local Community Nursing Services, this charity runs several nursing homes in different parts of the country. These provide hostel accommodation for patients receiving radiotherapy in a regional centre, short-stay admissions for pain control and other drug regimes to be established or stabilized, holiday admissions to give a break for relatives, and care for the terminally ill.

Details of local facilities may be obtained from:

> Marie Curie Foundation
> 124 Sloan Street
> London
> SW1X 9BP

or Marie Curie Foundation
> 21 Rutland Street
> Edinburgh
> EH1 2AE

Chest, Heart and Stroke Association

Patients with any chronic respiratory or cardiac condition may benefit from financial assistance towards fuel bills, fares, holidays etc., by application to the local branch or:

> Chest, Heart and Stroke Association
> Tavistock House North
> Tavistock Square
> London
> WC1H 9JE

Benevolent Societies

Patients who have served in the Forces and now need some financial assistance may be eligible for help from such bodies as the Solders, Sailors & Airmen's Families Association (SSAFA), the Earl Haig Fund or the RAF Benevolent Fund. If there is no local branch listed in the telephone directory, application may be made by the doctor or social worker to:

> SSAFA
> 16–18 Old Queen Street
> London
> SW1H 9HP

> Earl Haig Fund
> 48 Pall Mall
> London
> SW1Y 5JY

> RAF Benevolent Fund
> 67 Portland Place
> London
> W1N 4AR

CancerLink

This organization provides information and emotional support for people with cancer, their relatives and friends. In addition it publishes directories of useful organizations and cancer support groups throughout the United Kingdom.

CancerLink
46 Pentonville Road
London
N1 9HF

GINGERBREAD

This organization is more correctly termed:

Association for One Parent Families
35 Wellington Street
London WC2

Motor Neurone Disease Association

This association can offer financial advice and practical support, the details of local groups and publishes excellent leaflets to help the relatives.

Motor Neurone Disease Association
38 Hazelwood Road
Northampton
NN1 1LN

Multiple Sclerosis Society of Great Britain and Northern Ireland

286 Munster Road
Fulham
London
SW6 6AP

RUKBA

Royal United Kingdom Benificent Association (RUKBA)
6 Avonmore Road
London
W14 8RL

Samaritans Incorporated

This organization, offering telephone help or personal counselling, is so well known as to need no description. Details and addresses of the many branches throughout the country are obtainable from:

Samaritans Incorporated
17 Uxbridge Road
Slough
Berks
SL1 1SN

Registered Nursing Home Association

The details of all registered nursing homes in the UK may be
obtained from:

75 Portland Place
London
W1N 4AN

Appendix 3

GENERIC AND PROPRIETARY NAMES OF DRUGS COMMONLY USED IN TERMINAL CARE

acetylsalicylic acid	Aspirin, Disprin, Solprin
aminoglutethimide	Orimeten
aminophylline	Phyllocontin
amitriptyline	Lentizol, Triptizol
amphotericin B	Fungilin
baclofen	Lioresal
bendrofluazide	Neo-naclex
benorylate	Benoral
bisacodyl	Dulcolax
bromhexine	Bisolvon
bupivacaine	Marcain
buprenorphine	Temgesic
carbamazepine	Tegretol
chlordiazepoxide	Librium
chlormethiazole	Heminevrin
chlorpromazine	Largactil
chlorpropamide	Diabinese
cholestyramine	Questran
cimetidine	Tagamet
clobazam	Frisium
clomipramine	Anafranil
crotamiton	Eurax
cyclizine	Valoid
cyclophosphamide	Endoxana
dexamethasone	Decadron
dextromoramide	Palfium

dextropropoxyphene (and paracetamol)	Co-proxamol (Distalgesic)
diamorphine	Heroin
diazepam	Stesolid, Valium
dichloralphenazone	Welldorm
diflunisal	Dolobid
digoxin	Lanoxin
diphenoxylate	Lomotil
domperidone	Motilium
doxepin	Sinequan
emepronium	Cetiprin
ethamsylate	Dicynene
flurazepam	Dalmane
flurbiprofen	Froben
frusemide	Lasix
glibenclamide	Daonil
haloperidol	Serenace
hexamine hippurate	Hiprex
ibuprofen	Brufen, (Nurofen)
imipramine	Tofranil
indomethacin	Indocid
lactulose	Duphalac
loperamide	Imodium
lorazepam	Ativan
mebeverine	Colofac
medroxyprogesterone	Provera
mefenamic acid	Ponstan
metformin	Glucophage
methadone	Physeptone
methotrimeprazine	Nozinan, Veractil
methyldopa	Aldomet
methylprednisolone	Depo-medrone, Solu-medrone
metoclopramide	Maxolon, Gastrobid

mianserin	Bolvidon, Norval
morphine sulphate	M.S.T.
nefopam	Acupan
nitrazepam	Mogadon
nitrofurantoin	Furadantin
pericyazine	Neulactil
perphenazine	Fentazin
phenazocine	Narphen
phenytoin	Epanutin
piroxicam	Feldene
prochlorperazine	Stemetil
propantheline	Pro-banthine
propranolol	Inderal
ranitidine	Zantac
salbutamol	Ventolin
sodium phenobarbitone	Gardenal
sodium valproate	Epilim
spironolactone	Aldactone
tamoxifen	Nolvadex
temazepam	Normison
thiethylperazine	Torecan
thioridazine	Melleril
triamcinolone	Adcortyl
triazolam	Halcion
trimeprazine	Vallergan
trimipramine	Surmontil

Appendix 4

PATIENT'S PAIN RECORD (PPR)

Name of Patient: *Date of Birth:*

DATE	MORNING	EVENING
	No Pain ———————— Agony	No Pain ———————— Agony
	No Pain ———————— Agony	No Pain ———————— Agony
	No Pain ———————— Agony	No Pain ———————— Agony
	No Pain ———————— Agony	No Pain ———————— Agony
	No Pain ———————— Agony	No Pain ———————— Agony
	No Pain ———————— Agony	No Pain ———————— Agony
	No Pain ———————— Agony	No Pain ———————— Agony
	No Pain ———————— Agony	No Pain ———————— Agony
	No Pain ———————— Agony	No Pain ———————— Agony
	No Pain ———————— Agony	No Pain ———————— Agony
	No Pain ———————— Agony	No Pain ———————— Agony
	No Pain ———————— Agony	No Pain ———————— Agony
	No Pain ———————— Agony	No Pain ———————— Agony
	No Pain ———————— Agony	No Pain ———————— Agony

Notes for Patient
    (1) Complete at same time each morning and evening
    (2) Place a cross (X) on the point on the line which best describes the intensity of pain.

Appendix 5

BIBLIOGRAPHY

Comprehensive texts on Terminal Care (professional readers)

Chalmers G L 1980
Caring for the elderly sick. Pitman Medical, Tunbridge Wells
Doyle D (ed.) 1984
Palliative care: the management of far-advanced illness. Croom Helm, London
Martinson I M 1976
Home care for the dying child. Appleton-Century Crofts, New York
Saunders C 1984
The management of terminal malignant disease. Edward Arnold, London
Wilkes E 1982
The dying patient. MTP Press, Lancaster

Pain Control (professional readers)

Twycross R G Lack S A 1983
Symptom control in far-advanced cancer: pain relief. Pitman, London

Symptom Control (professional readers)

Twycross R G, Lack S A 1984
Therapeutics in terminal cancer. Pitman, London
Twycross R G, Lack S A 1986
Control of alimentary symptoms in far advanced cancer. Churchill Livingstone, Edinburgh

Spiritual problems (professional and lay readers)

Ainsworth-Smith I, Speck P 1983
Letting Go. SPCK, London
Fish S, Shelly J A 1978
Spiritual care. Inter Variety Press
Jacobs M 1982
Still small voice. SPCK, London
Lewis C S 1973
The problem of pain. Fontana Books
Neuberger J 1987
Caring for dying people of different faiths. Lisa Sainsbury Foundation, 8 Crown Hill, Croydon, Surrey CR0 1RY
Speck P 1978
Loss and grief in medicine Ballière Tindall, London

Psychological Needs of Patients, Relatives and Professionals

Stedeford A 1984
Facing death. William Heinemann, London
Lichter I 1987
Communication in cancer care. Churchill Livingstone, Edinburgh

Grief and Bereavement

Cathcart F 1984
In: Doyle D (ed.) Palliative care. Croom Helm, London
Hinton J 1972
Dying. Penguin Books, London
Kubler-Ross E 1970
On death and dying. Tavistock, London
Pincus, L 1976
Death and the family. Faber and Faber, London.
Torrie, M 1975
Begin again. J.M. Dent, London

For the Dying Patient

Casson J H
Dying: the greatest adventure of my life. Christian Medical Fellowship Publications, 157 Waterloo Road, London

For relatives of dying patients

Burton L 1974
Care of the child facing death. Routledge and Paul, London
Doyle D 1984
Coping with a dying relative. Chambers, Edinburgh

Grieving for a dead parent (for younger readers)

Krementz J 1983
How it feels when a parent dies. Victor Gollancz, London
William G, Ross J 1983
When people die. McDonald Publishers (Chambers), Edinburgh

Index